"Dr. Knowlton's book gives readers a blueprint and pathway towards healing by setting appropriate boundaries; purposeful sharing; expressions of empathy; and reclaiming authenticity and sexuality. This book has been needed in the field for a long time and is a must read for those who have survived relational betrayal through infidelity and problematic sexual behaviors."

James C. Wadley, *PhD, CST-S, Editor of* Leading Conversations about Black Sexualities and Identities

"Laney Knowlton has built her reputation on providing sensitive and supportive care to those struggling with problematic patterns of behavior and those healing from betrayal. Within these pages, she shares her wisdom; encouraging the reader to think expansively about what individual and relational health can look like, holding space for hurt without punishing the transgressor, and empowering each person to define what healing looks like for themselves and their relationship."

Stefani Goerlich, *PhD, LMSW-C, LISW, LCSW, CST*

"Dr. Laney Knowlton has masterfully written about the Connected Recovery Model which was developed to help individuals follow a guide for understanding what has happened to them regarding their betrayal, infidelity, and problematic sexual behaviors. *Healing from Betrayal, Infidelity, and Problematic Sexual Behaviors: A Guide to Individual and Relational Recovery* explains how this recovery should include both individual and relational recovery (if it applies). Dr. Knowlton exposes you to many exercises that have created profound changes in the recovery field. This model normalizes the confusion that naturally occurs when discovery occurs. It is as if she has joined your world and sees your fear, confusion, and trauma and she eloquently lays out a plan to assist you in your feelings and gives you hope that you will learn from your recovery and grow stronger as a result. This book is a must read for any individual who has been affected by problematic sexual behavior. This model invites you to work on yourself, your trauma, your shame and move towards your own personal resilience to find yourself perhaps for the very first time."

Carol Juergensen Sheets, *LCSW, CCES-S, CSAT-S, CCPS-S, CPC-S*

"*Healing from Betrayal, Infidelity, and Problematic Sexual Behaviors: A Guide to Individual and Relational Recovery* offers a clear, trauma-informed formula for helping readers heal from both problematic sexual behaviors and the resulting trauma experienced by their partners. With the sure-footedness of a seasoned guide leading wounded travelers through a wilderness of pain, Dr. Knowlton gently walks readers through a three-phase recovery journey – from inner despair to the discovery of a stronger, higher self."

Janice Caudill, *PhD, CSAT-S, CCPS-S, CPTT-S, PBTT, IAT, SEP*

Healing from Betrayal, Infidelity, and Problematic Sexual Behaviors

This compassionate and practical guide is designed to help individuals and those in relationships navigate the aftermath of problematic behavioral patterns, infidelity, and betrayal.

This book guides readers through the process of rebuilding emotional safety, creating deep, meaningful connections with themselves and others and a healthy connection to sexuality. Based in Attachment Theory, this book offers a structured three-phase recovery model that guides readers through Early Recovery (Repair), Middle Recovery (Reconnect), and Late Recovery (Restore). Chapters explore trauma and escape cycles, identifying relational dysfunction, emotional needs, breaking unhealthy behavioral patterns, restoring sexual connection, and staying grounded in the work of processing and healing. A chapter on parenting after betrayal is also included, which offers strategies for talking to your children and changing intergenerational patterns. This book puts evidence-based theory into practice through interactive tools including worksheets, diagrams, and exercises, helping readers hone boundary-setting skills, create individual and relationship check-ins, and more. Dr. Knowlton's sex-positive, inclusive, and non-shaming approach ensures concepts are accessible to all identities, sexualities, cultures, and relationship dynamics.

This comprehensive guide is essential to individuals and relationships struggling with infidelity and problematic behavioral patterns, as well as therapists looking to provide meaningful support to their clients.

Laney Knowlton, PhD, LMFT-S, CST, CSAT-S, CPTT-S, CCPS, CCRDS-S, CCBRT, RAE, specializes in PSB, infidelity, and betrayal. She has a Master's degree in marriage and family therapy and a PhD in clinical sexology.

Healing from Betrayal, Infidelity, and Problematic Sexual Behaviors

A Guide to Individual and Relational Recovery

Laney Knowlton

Routledge
Taylor & Francis Group

NEW YORK AND LONDON

Designed cover image: Getty Images

First published 2026
by Routledge
605 Third Avenue, New York, NY 10158

and by Routledge
4 Park Square, Milton Park, Abingdon, Oxon, OX14 4RN

Routledge is an imprint of the Taylor & Francis Group, an informa business

© 2026 Laney Knowlton

Library of Congress Cataloging-in-Publication Data
Names: Knowlton, Laney author
Title: Healing from betrayal, infidelity, and problematic sexual behaviors: a guide to individual and relational recovery / Laney Knowlton.
Description: New York, NY : Routledge, 2026. | Includes bibliographical references and index. |
Identifiers: LCCN 2025018764 (print) | LCCN 2025018765 (ebook) |
ISBN 9781041033370 hardback | ISBN 9781041033356 paperback |
ISBN 9781003623359 ebook
Subjects: LCSH: Sexual disorders—Treatment | Sex addiction |
Adultery | Couples—Psychology
Classification: LCC RC556 .K57 2026 (print) | LCC RC556 (ebook)
LC record available at https://lccn.loc.gov/2025018764
LC ebook record available at https://lccn.loc.gov/2025018765

ISBN: 978-1-041-03337-0 (hbk)
ISBN: 978-1-041-03335-6 (pbk)
ISBN: 978-1-003-62335-9 (ebk)

DOI: 10.4324/9781003623359

Typeset in Sabon
by codeMantra

To my very favorite people:
My husband, Rob, and my children, Megan, Kylie, Elizabeth, Jack, Eva, and Laura

And to my clients:
It has been an honor working with you. Thank you for letting me be part of your process.

Contents

Preface
What Is the Connected Recovery® Model?

This book explains the process of recovery and walks individuals (and relationships if you are in one) through each step of the process of recovering from problematic behavioral patterns, infidelity, and betrayal. It was written to be read by both those who are struggling with problematic behaviors or have betrayed themselves and others, and those who have been betrayed and are potentially healing from betrayal trauma. The approach used is the Connected Recovery® model, which connects tools and ideas from current leaders in the fields of problematic sexual behaviors, betrayal trauma, infidelity, sex therapy, and relational counseling.

This book walks you through early, middle, and late recovery. Early recovery focuses on helping you recover, find, see, and/or share the truth with yourself and those connected to you, or helps support you through the process of discovering and/or understanding the truth about someone you love. Middle recovery helps you deepen your connection to yourself and others and increases your ability to feel and express empathy, using classic relational therapy tools with a betrayal-sensitive lens. Late recovery walks you through healing the deepest wounds connected to betrayal; those related to sexuality. Finally, the last section helps parents know how to break the relational chains of dysfunctional and disconnecting patterns within the family structure and walks them through how to talk to their children (no matter what age the children are) about recovery and betrayal.

Acknowledgements

The development of the Connected Recovery® model and the creation of this book has been an amazing journey, and I am deeply grateful to those who have guided and supported me throughout this process.

I am deeply appreciative of Kimber Tower and Darien Wilson for their instrumental role in unifying the Connected Recovery® model into a cohesive whole. Thank you to Leanne Johnston as well for your contributions to formatting the material and helping me put the pieces of this book together. Each of you has been invaluable in shaping these concepts into a clear and accessible framework.

To my colleagues, mentors, and friends who have guided me throughout this process, your wisdom, feedback, and belief in me and in this work have made all the difference. Special thanks to Bret Livingston, Renée Breazeale, Pennie Carnes, Dr. Leslie Guditis, Dr. Mike Bishop, Dr. Carol Messmore, Dr. Janice Caudill, Karen Norwood, Dr. Barbara Steffens, Dr. Kervins Clement, Dr. Brian Martin, Dr. Dina Hijazi, Rev. Daniel Gowan, Dr. Gene Klassen, Jeanne Vattuone, Dan Drake, Carol Juergensen Sheets, Dr. Erica Sarr, Dr. Patrick Carnes, Dr. Shane Kraus, Randall McDaniel, Dr. Dan Rosen, Dr. James Wadley, Dr. Sylvia Rosenfeld, Michael Nee, Dr. Ricky Siegel, Dr. Pebble Kranz, Dr. Stefani Goerlich, Dr. Amanda Franklin, Rev. Chris and Jennifer Goers, Karen and Marty Christensen, David Ashburner, all those who have gone through the CR training, and the NT-SHP community.

Thank you so much to my clients and colleagues who have shared their experiences and perspectives, providing real-world insights that have enriched the depth and applicability of this model.

To my family, my husband, Rob, and my children, Megan, Kylie, Beth, Jack, Eva, and Laura, my adopted mom, Jojo Blake (and her husband Dan), my adopted son, Chris, and my in-laws, Lee and Susan Knowlton, thank you so much for your patience, encouragement, and support throughout this process. I never would have made it without you.

Finally, to those who will read this book, I hope these pages serve as a guide and help you find healing, peace, connection, and joy.

Introduction

All healing journeys start with hope, even if it's just a whisper of it. One of my friends, who has struggled with patterns of problematic behaviors, sent me the following message (they gave me permission to use it here) – "Hope is hard at the beginning. Sometimes you don't even want hope because of how much you hate yourself. You're so full of shame and guilt. You have to almost force yourself to face the fact that hope is an option, that you might deserve it eventually. Also, if it focuses on truth, you have a lot to face when it comes to truthfulness (or previous lack thereof)." Those who have been betrayed often struggle to feel hope as well. It can feel like the whole world has blown up and the idea of feeling peace and joy again seems impossible.

Whether you are struggling with patterns of problematic behaviors, infidelity, and/or betrayal and deception, or you are healing from betrayal, and perhaps dealing with betrayal trauma, taking the steps toward recovery can be terrifying. It's also often the only way forward if we want to feel hope, peace, connection, and joy again. Dealing with problematic sexual behaviors (PSB), patterns of escape cycles, infidelity, and betrayal trauma can be one of the most painful experiences we ever go through. It can feel like our lives and our hearts have been ripped apart. It may seem impossible to ever feel whole again. It isn't. You CAN heal from this, both individually and relationally.

Exercises are included in this book to help you personalize and internalize the tools provided. I recommend you get a separate notebook or create an electronic document where you can record your answers to the questions rather than just think about them. Find a way to keep those answers protected. If you use a notebook, buy a safe to keep it locked up. If you create an electronic document, password protect it – make sure to share the password with someone (your therapist, sponsor, friend, or group member, not your significant other) in case you forget it. Protecting your answers allows you the safety to answer the questions honestly and maximizes what you get from this information and these tools.

Exercise Intro–1:

1. What are you most afraid of regarding your recovery process?
2. What are your hopes for your recovery process?

DOI: 10.4324/9781003623359-1

Before we get started, I want to state that you are more than any label you may connect to. These labels might apply to things you have done or were done to you, or they might be attempts to explain what happened and why it happened. Some common labels I hear from clients include "cheater" or "sex addict" if they have betrayed or are struggling with PSB, or "betrayed partner" if they have been betrayed. Other labels try to encapsulate the way we feel about ourselves. Some examples of these include "broken," "sick," "damaged." Labels can be helpful sometimes to help us identify aspects of our lives that we need tools to help heal or change, but whatever labels you feel apply to you, recognize that you are much more than just those patterns or that experience. You are first and foremost a person, and you are worthy of being loved and loving others. You have value. You aren't just a label.

Understanding PSB

Understanding the behaviors that have hurt you or others, whether you struggle with them or you are impacted by someone else struggling with them, can help you to process and heal from them. Problematic behaviors happen on a continuum. Where we are on the continuum can help us to understand the level of help we need to change those patterns, or the boundaries we need to protect ourselves while someone else heals from those patterns.

All problematic patterns are unhealthy ways of coping at some level. Let's talk specifically about problematic patterns of sexual behavior. How do you know if you are struggling with PSB or if you are connected to someone who is? PSB, like other escape behaviors, occur on a continuum (see Figure 0.1).

I can't give you a list of "healthy sexual behaviors" because that list will be different for each person and each relationship. Healthy sexual behaviors are behaviors that align with your moral values, allow you to fulfill the commitments you've made to yourself or others, encourage growth, development, and well-being for you and others, ensure the safety and well-being of yourself and others, show respect to yourself and others, and strengthen congruency and authenticity. Using the above definition, sexual behaviors become problematic when they are misaligned with your moral values, break commitments you've made to yourself or others, harm you or others physically, emotionally, or psychologically, put your life or someone else's life at risk, violate others, or involve deception and/or lack of consent.

The term "sex/love addiction" is one that's frequently connected to PSB. There are conflicting schools of thought in the mental health field around that term. The current diagnosis related to PSB at an out-of-control level is "compulsive sexual behavior disorder" (CSBD), which is listed under impulse control disorders, not addictions (World Health Organization, n.d.). Current research has not shown that withdrawal symptoms are part

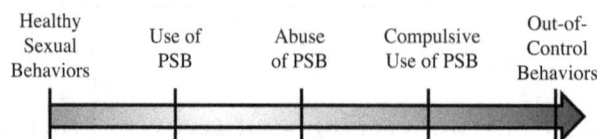

Healthy Sexual Behaviors	Use of PSB	Abuse of PSB	Compulsive Use of PSB	Out-of-Control Behaviors

Figure 0.1 Continuum of Problematic Sexual Behaviors

of the pattern. If studies show that stopping the behaviors cause withdrawal symptoms, it might be moved to the section that includes behavioral addictions. Either way, that is just the official label for the most extreme end of the continuum. The tools in the Connected Recovery® model work for any level of PSB.

If you fit the criteria for CSBD, you might initially need a higher level of care to change your patterns of behavior. CSBD might apply where there is a pattern of behavior (meaning it happens over and over) that you have been dealing with for six months or longer, have tried to stop multiple times but haven't been able to, which has caused significant problems for you and those connected to you. To qualify for the diagnosis, this pattern can't be the result of another mental health issue, like bipolar disorder or obsessive compulsive disorder, or the effect of substances or medications, or due to cognitive impairments, like Alzheimer's. If these behaviors are connected to another mental health issue, substances, or medications, you often still need help to change the patterns, but the treatment differs depending on the contributing factors. If you or someone you love fits these criteria, it doesn't mean you can't heal from the situation. It just helps understand the level of help needed at the beginning of the process.

Understanding Betrayal and Betrayal Trauma

Betrayal is a violation of a relational contract. This means that someone acts in a way that is opposite of what is expected, promised, or represented. The word has a lot of pain connected to it, so it applies to behaviors that are extreme enough to make those connected to the individual question their emotional safety within the relationship. It often includes secrecy and/or deception. Betrayal trauma is when the emotional and psychological impact of betrayal causes us to develop an attachment injury, which means being stuck in dysregulation. Not everyone who experiences betrayal develops betrayal trauma, but it is very common with romantic and sexual betrayal. Studies show that around two-thirds of those who experience betrayal in their primary relationships develop betrayal trauma (Hollenbeck & Steffens, 2024; Steffens & Rennie, 2006).

Betrayal trauma is similar to PTSD (Jules et al., 2023; Lonergan et al., 2021; Tirone et al., 2021). It can make it difficult to concentrate, cause you to have painful flashbacks, make it difficult to sleep because you're struggling with insomnia or nightmares, create situations where you significantly limit where you go and what you do because of fear of being reminded of the betrayal, create negative self-beliefs or beliefs about the world in general, make you lose interest in activities, isolate you, make it difficult to experience joy or happiness, cause you to develop hypervigilant behaviors, or make you irritable.

Whether or not you develop betrayal trauma as a result of experiencing betrayal, it is often incredibly painful to navigate. It is just as important for you to get help as for the person who has betrayed you to get help. If your symptoms are severe, a higher level of care might be helpful. Reaching out for help does not mean the betrayal is your fault. It isn't. I often have clients and clinicians ask something along the lines of, "What leads to being betrayed?" The answer is having someone violate the relational contract. It isn't not having enough sex, being a "co-addict," or being "codependent."

Exercise Intro–2:

1. What labels do you feel might connect to your path?
2. How do you feel about those labels?

There are many books and tools available that help walk you through the individual process of healing. Connected Recovery® is meant to be used in conjunction with individual programs. This book helps to combine individual recovery (connection to yourself) with relational recovery (connection to others) regardless of relational status, gender identity, or sexual orientation. Johann Hari (2015) said, "the opposite of addiction isn't sobriety, it's connection." While we aren't using the term "addiction," what I believe he meant was that unhealthy patterns and behaviors stem from a struggle to connect to others in healthy and meaningful ways. Trauma also disconnects us from ourselves and others. Healing at a deep level comes from processing through the things we've done and/or the things that have happened to us, creating a life where it is safe to connect with ourselves and others, and deepening that connection.

Connected Recovery® adds the connection piece to the recovery process, combining information from multiple organizations and trainings, including those in the field of treating PSB, infidelity, betrayal trauma, relational therapy, and sex therapy. I use similarities between the escape cycle and the trauma cycle (which I'll explain later) to build a foundation for connection and create a common language for those struggling with problematic patterns of behavior and those healing from betrayal. At the same time, I work hard to not minimize the pain those who have been betrayed go through or ignore the differences between the two paths. I am in no way saying that struggling with PSB and being betrayed are the same. This model provides tools that are helpful for both those struggling with PSB and those who have been betrayed and creates a common language that helps to create the potential for emotional safety, connection, and healing. It helps those who have been betrayed see and understand the work those struggling with problematic patterns are doing and helps those struggling with problematic patterns to gain a deeper understanding of the struggles and effort those they have hurt go through to heal. It also helps to ensure that trauma and attachment wounds are addressed for everyone connected to the situation.

Choosing a Therapist

I highly recommend starting the process by finding a therapist with specialized training. Find someone you feel comfortable with, who you feel safe talking to, and who seems to know what they're talking about. A good therapist will push you but will also help you feel hope.

Let me briefly explain the acronyms related to training in this area. IITAP (International Institute of Trauma and Addiction Professionals) offers several certifications, including CSAT, PSAP, CPTT, CCBRT, and RAE/RACS. Those with the CSAT (Certified Sex Addiction Therapist) are trained specifically to work with PSB at more extreme levels. PSAPs (Pastoral Sex Addiction Professionals) are also trained to work with PSB at more extreme levels, but from a religious approach. Professionals with either CSAT or PSAP credentials often use the term "sex addiction" and may not have training in working with betrayal, relationships, or providing sex therapy, especially if they went through their initial training years ago. The training program is working to incorporate more information about betrayal, relationships, and healthy sexual connection, but the focus is on treating "sex addiction." CPTTs (Certified Partner Trauma Therapists) are trained to work with those who have been betrayed. They may not have training to work with PSB, relationships, or healthy sexuality. CCBRTs (Certified Couples Betrayal Recovery Therapists) are trained to work specifically with the relationship in regards to betrayal. They often have some level of training related to working with PSB and/or betrayal, and may have some relational training. Those with RAE (Rainbow Advocate and Educator) and RACS (Rainbow Advocate Clinical Specialist) certifications are trained specifically to work with the LGBTQ+ population. They may or may not have training working with PSB or betrayal.

APSATS (Association of Partner of Sex Addicts Trauma Specialists) trains CCPSs (Certified Clinical Partner Specialists). Individuals with this certification are trained to work with those who have been betrayed. Both clinicians and coaches can get this certification. They may not have training to work with PSB, relationships, or healthy sexuality.

CSTs (Certified Sex Therapists) are often (but not always) certified through AASECT (American Association of Sex Educators, Counselors, and Therapists). They have training in healthy sexuality and sexual dysfunction. They may not have training in working with PSB, betrayal, or relationships.

SRWPs (Sexual and Relational Wellness Professionals) have training in healthy sexuality and relational dynamics. CFSs (Certified Forensic Sexologists) have the same foundational training as SRWPs, with additional training in PSB. These certifications are through SASH (Society for the Advancement of Sexual Health).

MFTs (Marriage and Family Therapists) have a master's or doctorate in Marriage and Family Therapy. The letters for this license differ by state. For example, in Texas, licensed MFTs are LMFTs, but in Kansas, they're called LCMFTs. Internationally, this license doesn't exist in many countries, so look for someone who specializes in relationships. Professionals in this area have training in working with relational dynamics. They often don't have training working with PSB, betrayal, or healthy sexuality.

There are additional programs that offer certifications in one or more of these four areas (PSB, betrayal, relationships, and healthy sexuality), but the ones listed above are the most commonly known.

If you're struggling with PSB, look for a CSAT (or CMAT if you are struggling with multiple co-occurring issues such as PSB and substance use) or PSAP (PSAPs are Pastoral Sex Addiction Professionals, so they can be helpful if you are looking for someone who will incorporate religious beliefs). There are also CSTs (Certified Sex Therapists) who specialize in PSB and betrayal. Additionally, many SRWPs or CFSs have specialized training in treating PSB and betrayal. You can google those letters, or you can go to IITAP.com to find a CSAT, CMAT, or PSAP, or to AASECT.org to find a CST. SRWPs and CFSs are listed at SASH.net. Many of those listed on the SASH website are connected to IITAP or AASECT.

If you are dealing with betrayal trauma, look for a CCPS or CPTT. You can google those letters or go to APSATS.org to find a CCPS, or IITAP.com to find a CPTT, or to AASECT.

org and look for someone who specializes in betrayal. SRWPs or CFSs may also specialize in betrayal; you can find those at SASH.net. Many of those on the SASH directory are also connected to IITAP, APSATS, or AASECT.

If you are LGBTQ+, kink, or poly, I highly recommend looking for a clinician who is trained specifically to work with LGBTQ+, kink, or poly folx. Look for a clinician who is a CST (Certified Sex Therapist) **and** specializes in PSB and/or betrayal recovery. I'd recommend starting with SASH.net or AASECT.org, although IITAP.com offers specialized training related to working with LGBTQ+ folx, so someone with a RAE (Rainbow Advocate and Educator) or RACS (Rainbow Advocate and Clinical Specialist) certification might be a good fit if you are LGBTQ+.

There are therapists who specialize in this area, but don't have outside certifications and training. I recommend finding one who has taken the steps to get professional training in these areas. Also, please note that, as with any profession, certifications in these fields don't guarantee that a therapist will be a good fit for you or that they are a good therapist. Pay attention to your gut. If it feels wrong (note that "wrong" is different than "uncomfortable" – a lot of therapeutic work is uncomfortable or even painful), find a different therapist.

Coaches specifically trained in this area can be helpful as well, especially when they work as a team with therapists. Coaches can help you work through the steps of recovery, but you will need to work with a therapist to process trauma connected to your experience and your recovery.

If you are going through this process in a relationship, I recommend finding a different individual therapist for each of you and highly recommend having each of your individual therapists communicate with each other around your recovery process. In early recovery, if your relationship includes two people, I recommend using a cotherapy format for couples' work, meaning both individual therapists are in the room for a couple's session. This is more difficult if you have more than two people in the relationship, so if your relationship includes more than two people, I recommend individual therapists for each of you and a relational counselor for your relational work.

There are several reasons I recommend using cotherapy if possible. While this is more expensive, it makes the process much faster and easier. You each know you have someone in the room to support you, so you don't have to worry about it feeling like the therapist is on one person's side. You don't have to waste time explaining what happened in your relational session to your individual therapist. And you have someone in the room who knows you and can call you on your "stuff" as it happens and provide support in an individualized way. Additionally, if you experience strong emotions in the session, you can split up and process your emotions in the moment instead of having to either wait for an individual session or have the relational therapist take turns processing with one of you while the other waits outside. Once you've gotten into middle recovery and have a strong foundation of trust built in the relationship, you can switch to using a third therapist as your relational therapist if you prefer. Don't use one of your individual therapists as the relational therapist. If one of you has an individual relationship with the therapist, it will likely be very difficult for the sessions to feel balanced and each of you to feel supported, no matter how good the therapist is at being neutral.

Exercise Intro–3:

1. Do you have an individual therapist? If not, what steps might be helpful for you to find one?
2. If you are in a primary relationship, do you have a relational counselor? If not, what steps might be helpful for you to find one?

Group Therapy

Group therapy is an important tool in recovery. Groups help connect you to others who are going through similar struggles. They help you know you aren't alone, connect you to others you can be honest with about your struggles and experience, and help you learn tools others have developed to deal with similar issues.

There are several different types of groups. Each type provides something different. Some of these tools will be helpful for you and others might not be. If possible, I recommend joining a group led by a therapist or therapists. Some groups, called process groups, are on-going. These are often smaller (my groups max out at eight participants) and offer you the chance to form long-term friendships and connections with other group members. Others are limited to a specific time (6 weeks, 8 weeks, 12 weeks, etc.) and usually have a specific format they follow or topic they focus on, allowing you to learn with, and from, others about that topic. Groups led by therapists usually give you a chance to process through issues you're dealing with, interact with others during group (12 step groups usually don't allow "cross-talk" as they are led by peers, not therapists), and offer recovery tools.

Recovery coaches often offer groups as well. Groups run by recovery coaches should not offer trauma processing but provide tools to help you in your healing process and allow you to connect with others dealing with similar situations. They may be long-term or for a limited time. Coaches can offer services across state lines, so these groups are often virtual and offer services to a larger area.

There are very few therapist- or coach-led groups that are geared toward LGBTQ+ folx struggling with PSB or recovering from betrayal. I am not aware of any that specifically advertise as kink or poly friendly groups. If you are looking for a group that is LGBTQ+, kink, or poly friendly, I recommend looking for clinicians who are CSTs, SRWPs, or CFSs **and** running groups for PSB or betrayal recovery. The therapist may have other trainings as well, but a professional with one of those certifications are much more likely to understand more about LGBTQ+, kink, and poly issues. Contact the professional and talk with them about whether or not their group might be a good fit for you. Trust your instincts. If you don't feel comfortable with them, chances are you will not feel comfortable in their group.

Additionally, if you are struggling with problematic patterns of behavior, 12 step groups are available in person and virtually. The language used in 12 step groups is outdated and some of the groups are rigid and shaming, but there are many groups that are helpful and supportive. They are free and often have meetings multiple times a week. Twelve step groups focus on avoidance of unhealthy behaviors (sobriety) and provide peer support. As they are led by peers, they do not offer processing and the tools they offer are those that have worked for the specific people you are connected to, rather than generalized therapeutic tools. If this type of group seems like it might be helpful for you, I encourage you to visit a few 12 step groups and see if you can find one that you feel comfortable with.

There are three major 12 step groups for PSB. These groups use the terms "sex addiction" and "love addiction." Whether or not you connect to that term, 12 step groups can provide peer support and help you work toward stopping behaviors you're struggling with. SAA (Sex Addicts Anonymous) focuses on avoiding "selfish sex" and is probably the most used ministry for males struggling with PSB. It is relatively easy to find "male only" SAA meetings. SLAA (Sex and Love Addicts Anonymous) is the only ministry to include "love addiction" (problematic behaviors related to romantic fantasy preoccupation) as well as "sex addiction" and is most frequently used by females struggling with PSB. It is easier to find "female only" meetings through SLAA as opposed to other 12 step groups. There are specific SAA and SLAA groups geared toward LGBTQ+ folx and some groups are inclusive and welcoming even if they don't advertise as specifically being LGBTQ+ friendly. Some SLAA groups and a few SAA groups are kink or poly friendly. Internet searches can provide a list of groups that advertise as inclusive. SA (Sexaholics Anonymous) is the strictest regarding definitions and has the strongest religious undertones, defining sexual sobriety as sex within a heterosexual marriage, and focuses on avoiding "lust."

Twelve steps groups are available for those who have been betrayed, too. Like the 12 step groups for those struggling with PSB, they use language that was originally developed when the field started, like "sex addiction," "codependent," and "betrayed partner." S-Anon, COSA (Codependents of Sex Addicts), CoDA (Codependents Anonymous), ISA (Infidelity Survivors Anonymous) and Al-Anon are all groups that clients I've worked with who have been betrayed have found helpful. The vast majority of these groups primarily include heterosexual women who have been betrayed. Al-Anon is the easiest to find an LGBTQ+ friendly group through. It is more difficult to find groups focused on betrayal recovery that advertise as kink or poly friendly. Most groups say they are inclusive, but poly and kink clients I've worked with have struggled to find groups in which they felt comfortable openly disclosing those aspects of their relationships. Keep in mind that most of them were named when the field still referred to those who have been betrayed as either "co-addicts" or "codependent." Despite the names being outdated, these groups can sometimes provide very helpful, low-cost support for those who have been betrayed. As I mentioned earlier, if this tool seems like it might be helpful for you, I encourage you to visit a few 12 step groups and see if you can find one that you feel comfortable with.

Exercise Intro—4:

1. What groups are you already part of?
2. What additional groups, if any, might be helpful for you to explore? What steps will you take to do so?

Emotional Bucket Filling

As you go into this process, there are a few essential pieces of the puzzle that are helpful to add at the beginning. I define recovery as becoming whole, connecting to yourself and to others and healing from the things you've experienced, either because of your own actions or the actions of others, usually some combination of both. Connection to self and others fills our emotional "bucket," and we need a combination of connection to self and others in order to fill our bucket. In general, half of your bucket needs to be filled with connection to self and half needs to be filled with connection to others. The specifics as to what fills your bucket will be different for each person. There are four basic categories that bucket-fillers fall into: excitement, creativity, relaxation, and connection. Again, the activities in each of these categories are very individual. What's exciting for one person may be relaxing for another person or may not be a bucket-filler at all.

Connection to Others – Building a Support System

You can't do this on your own. You need support and connection. Your therapist(s) and group(s) can be an important part of your support system. I call it a superhero squad – you're welcome to use that term, come up with your own term, or just call them your support system. In general, you need a minimum of five people on your superhero squad. It's unlikely that any one person will be able to provide you with support in every area you need support in, but make sure to have 2–3 members of your squad that you can talk to about each major part of your life. These areas can overlap. For example, you might need support around what you're going through with your behaviors or your significant other's behaviors. You might need support around how this affects your children. You might need support around your job. Let's say your squad includes Jaime, Pat, Sam, Jodie, and Alex. Maybe Jaime, Sam, and Jodie are the members of your squad you can reach out to for support around the PSB/betrayal, Pat and Sam can give you support related to your children, and Pat, Jodie, and Alex can give you support related to your job.

You need some connection to others every day, even if it's just a text or a phone call. At least once a week, find some activity you can do with at least one other person that takes at least an hour.

Exercise Intro–5:

1. What are the primary areas of your life you might need support around?
2. Who can you add to your superhero squad?

Connection to Self – Rediscovering Joy

One of the first exercises I have my clients do is start adding in "bucket-fillers," or things that bring them joy. This is the beginning of connecting to yourself. I recommend spending five minutes each day doing something that brings you joy, and once a week doing something that takes at least an hour that brings you joy. Often these things are seen as "childish" or "silly." I don't care if it's child-like or silly – if it brings you joy, it's worth doing. Focus on things that are related to your senses: things you see, touch, taste, smell, or hear. I've had clients who stopped to watched the sunrise or sunset, got a corn dog at Sonic, treated themselves to their favorite specialized coffee or drink, stopped and watched roly-polies on the sidewalk, bought hand soap in their favorite scent, kept Dove chocolates in their desk or purse, watched birds eating fish, had soft blankets tucked away in their offices or homes, listened to recorded sounds of the ocean or rainstorms, or had playlists of their favorite songs divided by emotion or situation.

Beyond learning the "little" things you enjoy, recognize that each of us needs excitement, relaxation, creativity, and connection. Things that are exciting for us raise our energy levels; those that are relaxing calm our energy levels. Creativity adds color to our lives and makes something new. Connection strengthens your relationships with yourself and others. As long as the behaviors don't harm you or others (physically, emotionally, or psychologically), the sky's the limit! Work to not judge yourself for the activities you choose and to figure out activities that actually meet each need for you. Many of my clients initially only consider ideas that meet the generally accepted "norms" for each category, but they might meet different needs for you than what you expect. For example, rock-climbing might be exciting for one person, relaxing for another, and terrifying for someone else. Crocheting might be exciting or relaxing, and add creativity to someone's life, while others might find it boring. Creating spreadsheets or organizing your home might be exciting and creative for one person and a drain for another. An important part of this exercise is learning to know yourself and how to meet your needs. If you need ideas, talk to your therapist and/or group, or other members of your support system. Some of your ideas might fit more than one category. For example, maybe going for a hike or bike ride is exciting or relaxing, and connecting if you go with a friend or if it gives you time to think and connect with yourself.

Exercise Intro–6:

1. What are five ideas for bucket-fillers that would add excitement to your life? Consider each of the senses as you come up with ideas. Make sure to think of ideas that would take less than five minutes and ones that would take at least an hour.

2. What are five ideas for bucket-fillers that would add relaxation to your life? Again, consider each of the senses as you come up with ideas and make sure to think of ideas that would take less than five minutes and ones that would take at least an hour.

3. Explore what creativity feels like to you and come up with at least five things that make you feel creative. Some people love activities that are traditionally viewed as creative, such as art, music, or writing. Others might enjoy organizing or running a business or marketing.

4. Back to the section on Connection to Others, what are some ideas of activities you could do that would make you feel connected to someone else? Come up with at least five things.

5. What are five activities that let you connect better to yourself? These often allow for introspection or deeper emotions (happiness, sadness, etc.).

Stages of Recovery

Recovery from PSB and/or betrayal is a process that takes about 3–5 years. That doesn't mean that you will be in the pain you are in currently for that whole time. It also doesn't mean that you or your primary partner(s) will magically shift into strong recovery/healing after that point if you or they don't do the work connected to it. It means that it takes about 3–5 years to process through the different phases of recovery, build a strong foundation, rebuild trust and safety, and get to a point where you have a strong connection to yourself and others and have healed from what you've gone through on the deepest levels.

I divide the recovery process into three phases: early, middle, and late recovery. In his Trust Revival Method (the process he developed to help couples recover from affairs), Gottman states that couples go through three phases to heal connection when there has been a betrayal; Atone, Attune, and Attach (Gottman & Silver, 2012). The first phase includes the individual who betrayed taking accountability for what they did, making amends, and working to repair the breach of trust. The second phase focuses on building a new relationship. The third and final phase deepens the connection by focusing on physical intimacy. I've combined elements from those three phases with Maslow's Hierarchy of Needs, as viewed through the lens of the steps from the Intimacy Pyramid (Caudill & Drake, 2020) to define the work in each phase of recovery. Combining the two incorporates individual healing into the relational process and provides additional tools to address patterns of betrayal as well as isolated betrayals, along with potential historical contributors (family-of-origin work, past traumas, attachment wounds from childhood and/or adolescence, etc.) to the development of the betrayal. Phase 1, Repair, works to Establish Truth and create Emotional Safety (this takes about 1–2 years). Phase 2, Reconnect, focuses on building Empathy and Connection (this takes about 1–2 years). Phase 3, Restore, concentrates on healing at the deepest levels through Healing Sexuality (this takes about a year).

Each phase of the Connected Recovery® model includes five components: Education, Honesty, Boundaries, Communication, and Connection. These components apply to anyone going through the recovery process, including those struggling with PSB and those healing from betrayal. As stated earlier, I am in no way saying that those who have been betrayed are "codependent," or that they did anything to contribute to the PSB or betrayal, or that they deserved to be betrayed. Rather, I'm stating that all of us have trauma cycles and all of us have some level of escape cycles (which can become extreme) and we can benefit by identifying and processing through those. Additionally, using the same tools creates a foundation for connection and allows the work that is done by both sides to be seen and understood by each other, helping to build trust and create safety.

While the similarities can be used to create a common language that every human being can connect to, there are some major differences in the process needed to heal escape patterns as opposed to those needed to heal from being betrayed. Those differences are addressed in the individual healing process each person goes through, which is one of the reasons why it's important to work with a clinician who specializes in either PSB or betrayal, depending on what you're going through. Although understanding the differences is essential, I have found that the differences in individual processes make it difficult for the person who has been betrayed to be able to see the work the person struggling with PSB is doing (or not doing if they choose not to work on their recovery) and for the person struggling with PSB to see and understand the pain their significant other or others are going through and the work their significant other or others are doing to heal. By having each individual go through the same process, each can see and understand the actions that are being taken. This creates safety for each and a foundation upon which trust can be rebuilt. It also makes it easier to connect in middle recovery (Phase 2) once it's safe to do so.

This book focuses on all three phases of Connected Recovery®, covering early, middle, and late recovery tools. It is written so both those struggling with PSB and those who have been betrayed can use the same book and speak the same language. It has tools that can help the individual recovery process, but additional steps are often helpful. This model works well in conjunction with individual recovery plans and helps to create a foundation for connection and to add relational work to the process. You can use the tools included in this book to explain your recovery work to each other and to rebuild your relationship and/or connection to others. If you are going into this process in a relationship, please note that you can heal whether or not your significant other(s) chooses to take the steps to work through recovery.

I define recovery as finding your whole self; figuring out who you are and who you want to be, healing from the wounds and patterns that affect your ability to be that person and discovering how to feel joy and peace again. You can find healing no matter where you are starting the process from, what's happened to you, or what you've done.

Exercise Intro–7:

1. What stood out to you as you read the introduction?
2. What questions do you have about the recovery process? Discuss those questions with your therapist and/or group.

Super Short Summary:

Problematic sexual behaviors (PSB) are sexual or romantic behaviors that cause pain to you and/or others in your life. Betrayal is a violation of a relational contract. Betrayal trauma is an attachment wound created by the violation of a relational contract. Find trained professionals to help you through the process of healing. Start by building a support system and adding little bits of joy to your life. It takes time, but healing is possible.

Chapter Questions:

1. What did you connect to the most in this chapter?
2. What steps are you taking to apply this material to your life?

Repair – Creating Emotional Safety Through Truth

Education

Understanding Trauma and Escape Cycles

Early recovery (Phase 1) focuses on creating emotional safety for yourself and others through truth. The first component in each phase of recovery is education. In early recovery, education focuses on understanding trauma and escape cycles. Let's start by exploring how dysfunction and escape patterns impact relationships. Keep reading even if you're single because we all have relationships with others and connection to others is an important part of recovery.

Every relationship (marriage or primary relationship, friendship, parent–child, sibling, etc.) is a connection between two or more. Each of those people is human. As human beings, we each have things we've learned, experiences we've gone through, and personality traits we have. These each contribute to the way we connect to others. Some of those traits and approaches are functional, meaning they increase our ability to connect to ourselves and others. Some are dysfunctional, meaning they create disconnection from ourselves and from others. Those we connect to tend to have about the same level of function/dysfunction as we do (this does not include escape patterns, abuse, or deception – we'll get to that in a minute).

There are some types of dysfunction that cause enough pain and harm to the system and those connected to it that that type of dysfunction needs to be addressed before we address the relational dysfunction. These behaviors fall into three categories: abuse, significant deception, and significant escape cycles. Betrayal can fall into all three categories. Those types of disconnecting behaviors make connection unsafe and can sabotage the relational work if they aren't addressed at the beginning of the process.

Because of the damage escape patterns, deception, and abuse cause, the earliest work in recovery focuses on creating safety. Those who have been betrayed start by working to create safety for themselves (because relying on the person who has betrayed them isn't safe at this point). Those struggling with problematic sexual behaviors start with learning to stop their behaviors and create safety for themselves. By the same token, in cases where there is abuse, the abuser needs to stop their behaviors and create safety for themselves and those connected to them, and the person being abused needs to start by creating safety for themselves, so their safety isn't based on the abuser protecting them because that isn't safe to rely on yet. Once we've taken those steps and built healthier and more helpful patterns, we can work on the dysfunctional patterns in the relationship and work to deepen connection to ourselves and others. That work happens in middle and late recovery (Phases 2 and 3).

DOI: 10.4324/9781003623359-3

Trauma

Let's start by talking about trauma. Trauma is an event or circumstance that results in physical, emotional, or life-threatening harm that has lasting effects on the individual's physical, emotional, psychological, and/or spiritual health or well-being (SAMHSA, 2024). The word trauma is often overused. Referring to the conversation we had in the introduction about betrayal and betrayal trauma, trauma indicates unresolved pain, not just a painful experience.

The extent of the effect of the trauma we experience is often directly related to the support we get regarding the situation. For example, being sexually assaulted is made worse when others connected to the person who was assaulted minimize or dismiss what happened or blame them for the assault. Another example might be betrayal trauma made worse by the person who betrayed continuing to lie about what happened or continuing to gaslight their significant other or others.

Judith Herman was one of the first to explain trauma in the terms listed above. Although her work was originally published in 1992, it has been supported and expanded and is still considered foundational for those who focus on understanding and treating trauma. Her work is the underlying model that the Multi-Dimensional Trauma Treatment model, the model APSATS uses to train clinicians and coaches, is based on. One of the underlying issues she identified was that trauma doesn't just come from the pain but comes from the fear that we will not be able to stop ourselves from continuing to be harmed. That fear makes us hyperalert, constantly watching out for additional situations that will harm us. Part of that hyperawareness is intrusive thoughts. Our brain brings up what we have gone through over and over again to try and make sense of what we went through. Because we are constantly on alert, we are mentally and emotionally exhausted and start avoiding things that might make our hyperawareness worse.

There are several types of trauma. Trauma can also be a combination of several types. Considering the types of trauma helps us to better understand the pain we've experienced that is still impacting our lives.

Historical/intergenerational trauma cycles are developed as a response to experiences or patterns that our ancestors lived through, the effects of which may still be felt, which are passed down to future generations. These traumas include experiences that have widespread effects, cause collective suffering, and include malicious intent (APA, 2022). Examples of this type of trauma include racism, the Holocaust, and Japanese American internment camps.

Interpersonal traumas involve emotional or physical neglect, and emotional, physical, or sexual abuse in childhood or adulthood (Mauritz et al., 2013). This type of trauma includes experiences such as being bullied, patterns of abuse or neglect, rejection, being gossiped about, or being excluded. The effect of these traumas often shows up in our current life even when current patterns or experiences are different. For example, if one of your parents used your weaknesses to manipulate you, you might have a trauma response when a significant other sees a weakness in you. This response may be completely unrelated to your significant other, meaning your significant other may not use your weaknesses to manipulate you. It's a pattern that you've learned to expect, so you've developed an automatic reaction to it.

Single-incident traumas are single terrible, harmful, or threatening events. Traumas in this category might include the death of a loved one, rape, a car accident, assault, or being mugged.

Vicarious trauma is pain and/or fear resulting from hearing about or becoming witness to someone else's pain, fear, or terror (Evces, 2015). This can be connected to historical/intergenerational trauma. It can also be connected to supporting someone else through a traumatic experience, such as listening to a friend process a traumatic experience. It's often identified in first responders, caregivers, medical professionals, and mental health professionals.

Physical/medical trauma relates directly to physical harm or damage to your body. In some cases, it might include physical attacks or injuries from an accident. In other situations, the damage might be an attempt to help your body heal, such as surgery. Surgery damages your body in one way in an attempt to repair it in another way. Even if the physical trauma is planned (such as surgery), and even if you ultimately benefit physically from the experience, the experience can cause lasting emotional trauma.

Betrayal trauma originates from significant violations of a person's trust or well-being by a trusted, needed other (Freyd, 2021). Betrayal trauma includes infidelity (both isolated events and patterns of behavior), institutional betrayal, or abuse by a caregiver. This also includes failure by a caregiver or institution (including religious organizations, societies, schools, medical facilities, etc.) to protect someone in their care. Betrayal trauma differs from other types of traumas, as survival often depends on continued interaction with the individual who betrayed you. Like other traumas, betrayal trauma means your world isn't safe anymore, but the dynamics connected to betrayal trauma often make recovery from the trauma more complex. For example, in the case of infidelity, often those who have been betrayed are linked to the person who betrayed them financially, or they have children together and therefore will need to coparent for the rest of their lives.

Exercise 1–1:

1. Which types of trauma have you experienced?
2. Which types of trauma do you think your significant other(s) or those in close connection to you have experienced?
3. What emotions and thoughts came up for you as you learned about the various types of trauma and considered how trauma might have influenced your life and the lives of those around you? Process your emotions and thoughts with your therapist and/or group.

The Trauma Cycle

Each of us has trauma cycles. Some of our trauma cycles are related to well-developed patterns, either patterns we are currently part of or patterns we became used to in previous relationships/situations. Some of our trauma cycles are responses to current situations. Some are a combination of both.

When we hit a point where our pain is too much to process, we automatically shift into a trauma cycle. Sometimes that's because the pain of a specific experience is too much to handle. Other times it's more of "the straw that broke the camel's back" and something that seems little pushes us over the edge into things being too much to deal with. Either way, we shift into survival responses. If the survival response doesn't resolve the situation immediately, we can stay stuck spinning in that response. It might make us temporarily feel like we are doing something about the situation, but survival responses only resolve imminent threats, so they don't fix traumas. Part of us realizes that and the realization makes us feel more powerless, which makes the initial pain feel even worse, and we stay stuck spinning in that cycle.

Exercise 1–2:

1. Can you identify a time when you shifted into a trauma cycle? What triggered this and how did you respond?
2. When you experience stress or trauma, can you tell whether your reaction is based on past trauma or the current situation? How can you tell what your reaction is based on?

Survival Responses

Survival mode shifts us into a different part of our brain called the limbic system. The limbic system does not function rationally, it functions reactively. If we hear a loud noise, we startle. If we're chased by a bear, we run. If we see something moving quickly toward us, we duck. Those are all examples of survival responses. We usually learn our survival responses in childhood, although abuse and very painful experiences at any point in life can create them as well.

Most people are familiar with the fight, flight, and freeze responses. Fight is when we actively fight against something we feel is threatening (remember, we're just talking about reactive responses in this case, not long-term decisions). Flight is when we run away from it. Freeze is when we stop moving and hope we blend into the background, like a deer in the woods when it hears a sound. It's important to recognize that our responses may have been learned in childhood, but they often look a little different in adulthood. Flight in childhood might be hiding behind a couch or in a closet so you won't be noticed. As an adult, it might look more like leaving the room, or dissociating, or checking out from a conversation.

I've found it helpful to include three additional responses: frenzy, fold, and fawn. These six seem to be those my clients most connect to. Frenzy, fold, and fawn aren't quite as well known. Frenzy is when we respond to threats by running around, looking like we're doing something, in an attempt to distract or deflect. This might happen if you hear the garage door open and know that you'll get yelled at if you are sitting and watching TV, so you jump up and start cleaning something, even if the room is completely clean. Fold is giving up and giving in. You don't believe anything you do will matter or make a difference in the situation, and so you just do what they tell you to do. Fawn is when you work to do everything you can for someone to keep them from getting mad or leaving or hurting you or someone else. It's not done because you're taking care of them in a connective way; it's done out of fear, often terror.

We are born with or develop survival responses because they work. They help us survive painful or dangerous parts of our life and often develop in childhood. Unless the situation is a life-or-death situation, our initial survival response doesn't resolve the situation. In cases where survival responses don't resolve the situation, we move to safe-harboring behaviors.

Exercise 1–3:

1. When faced with stress or conflict, which survival response (fight, flight, freeze, frenzy, fold, or fawn) do you tend to use most often? Why do you think this is?
2. Are there specific situations or people that tend to trigger a survival response in you? How do those situations make you feel afterward?
3. Survival responses develop because they work in the short term. How might you acknowledge the way your responses have protected you while also working toward healthier ways of coping?

Safe-Harboring

Survival responses work to protect us from imminent harm. If we have a car coming toward us and we jump backwards, the reflexive response works. We don't get hit by the car. Shifting into survival responses doesn't just happen when reactive responses would fix the situation. They happen when our brain and heart feel threatened. If that threat is emotional, reactive responses don't fix the situation. In those cases, we can stay trapped spinning in the survival response because our brains keep trying to fix the situation by responding reactively. I call that safe-harboring.

I grew up on Cape Cod and love the ocean. The ocean can be dangerous though. If you are caught on a boat in the middle of a storm, you need to find a safe harbor that provides protection in order to survive the storm. Similarly, if you are in the middle of a trauma response, you automatically work to create safety, so you survive. You will likely look for "safe harbors" that have previously helped you weather storms and use techniques that have kept your boat afloat in other storms. The issue with these patterns is that we've outgrown those harbors and they don't help resolve situations.

Safe-harboring behaviors fall into three general categories: mirror, shield, and sword. (See Figure 1.1.)

Mirror responses correlate to freeze or fold survival responses. Both freeze and fold abdicate our ability to control situations. We can't move, we can't make decisions, we give up on trying to elicit change and believe the only way to create safety is to rely on someone else to change. This often comes from being taught that we aren't allowed to create safety or that any attempts on our part to create safety will fail. I use the term "mirror" because when we're spinning in these responses, we are immobilized, and we reflect the ability to create safety onto others. Examples of mirror responses include acting like nothing happened or shutting down. Freeze and fold look the same externally, but they feel completely opposite. In a freeze response, our nervous system is on high alert. In a fold response, our nervous system shuts down.

Shield responses try to create safety by minimizing reactivity in ourselves and others, minimizing consequences for others and therefore ourselves, and reducing chaos. The survival responses connected to shielding are fawn and frenzy. These survival responses focus on buffering others with the idea that focusing on calming others down or providing distractions will create safety. Examples of shield responses might be exaggerating all the good things someone that hurt them has done and not addressing the pain they are feeling, or pretending some hurtful or painful comment someone else made was a joke.

Sword responses are coupled with fight and flight. Both fight and flight are active reactions. Fight involves staying in the situation and escalating to attempt to create safety. Flight might look like a passive response, but it is actively working to change the situation by escaping it. Examples of sword responses include yelling or threatening (not stating boundaries – that's not threatening someone, even if others perceive boundaries as threats – we'll talk about that later) or leaving the room to shut down a conversation instead of processing it.

All three types of safe-harboring only work short-term. These responses are often incongruent with who we want to be, don't actually create safety, and cause disconnection from ourselves and others.

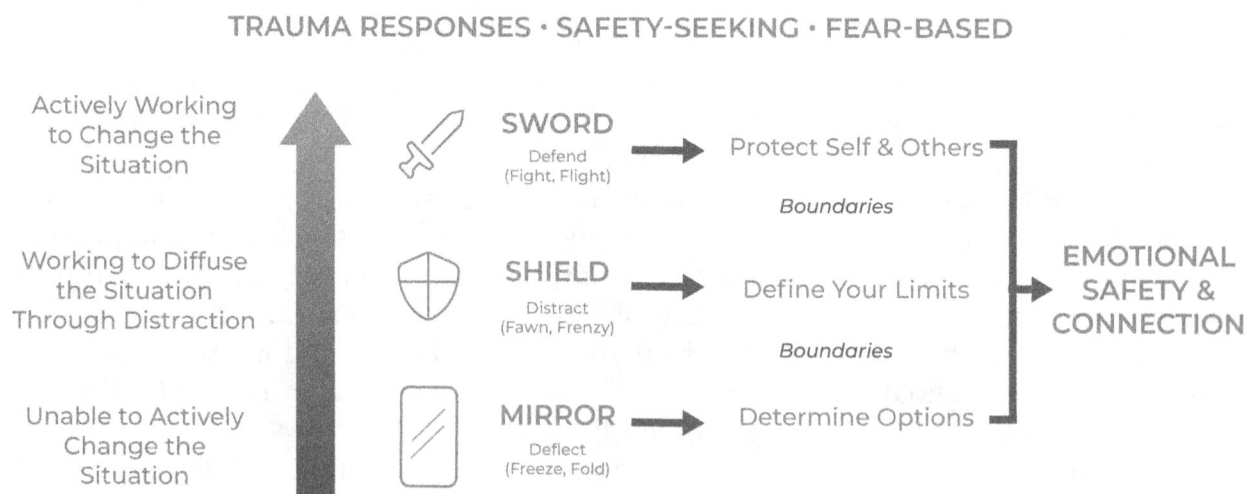

TRAUMA RESPONSES · SAFETY-SEEKING · FEAR-BASED

Actively Working to Change the Situation

SWORD
Defend
(Fight, Flight)

→ Protect Self & Others

Boundaries

Working to Diffuse the Situation Through Distraction

SHIELD
Distract
(Fawn, Frenzy)

→ Define Your Limits

Boundaries

Unable to Actively Change the Situation

MIRROR
Deflect
(Freeze, Fold)

→ Determine Options

EMOTIONAL SAFETY & CONNECTION

Figure 1.1 **Levels of Safe-Harboring Responses**

Exercise 1–4:

1. When you feel emotionally threatened, do you tend to respond with a mirror, shield, or sword response? Why do you think this is?
2. Because safe-harboring only works in the short term, what is one small step you can take to begin responding in a way that fosters real safety and connection rather than temporary relief?

Your Trauma Cycle

The worksheet in Figure 1.4 (My Trauma Cycle) helps walk you through understanding why something hurt you and what you can do to heal from it. Briefly, starting on the left of the worksheet, we have a painful experience. When that experience is unresolved, meaning if it is too big to resolve without additional steps or within our current system, or if there is too much to process and it overwhelms us, we shift into the trauma cycle. The trauma cycle is represented by the box and expanded in the area to the right of the box. The different types of trauma are listed in the box to help you consider all contributing factors that created the unresolved pain. The circle of arrows starts with identifying your initial survival response, followed by your safe-harboring response. This might be the same as your initial survival response or it might be different. For example, maybe your initial response is to freeze, then you shift into a shield response, distracting from the situation to attempt to diffuse it. Everything we do makes sense in context. Safe-harboring responses work short term, which is why we do them. Identify how your response impacted the situation under "temporary benefit." They don't work long term though. They make us feel worse and don't resolve the situation. Write down the way the safe-harboring response impacts you and the situation long term under "long-term consequences."

Because trauma comes from pain we are unable to resolve, the way out of the trauma cycle involves working to process through what we experienced. The arrows out of the box that lead across the top are the steps to process through the experience. The first step is to vent or soothe. Venting is letting energy out. Soothing is calming energy down. Both relieve some of the emotional pressure. Make sure not to vent to the person you have been upset by and don't look to them to help soothe you. This is one of the reasons it's important to have at least five people in your support system. Decreasing the energy helps you to be able to see the underlying cause of the pain more clearly. First consider the emotions you're feeling. Use the emotions chart in Figure 1.2 and focus on the outer circle. It's ok to include some of the words in the inner circle, but they are too general to identify your needs. Core emotions are the equivalent of telling a doctor "I hurt." The doctor needs more information to understand what's going on, just as you need more specific emotions to process the experience. Once you have identified the emotions, look at the Hierarchy of Needs chart (Figure 1.3). When asked what we need, usually people respond with solutions, not needs. Solutions are actions we take, or we ask others to take to meet our needs. Identifying the need can help understand which solutions might be most helpful. Potential solutions can be entered under "how to meet need" on the worksheet. Make sure at least one or two of the solutions are ones that you can implement yourself. You can still ask others, such as the person involved in the situation that triggered you, to make changes, but you need options that create safety for yourself if they are unwilling or unable to make those changes.

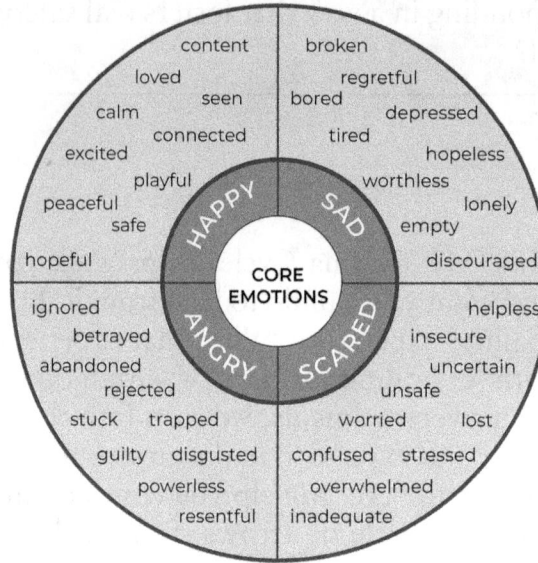

Figure 1.2 Emotions Chart

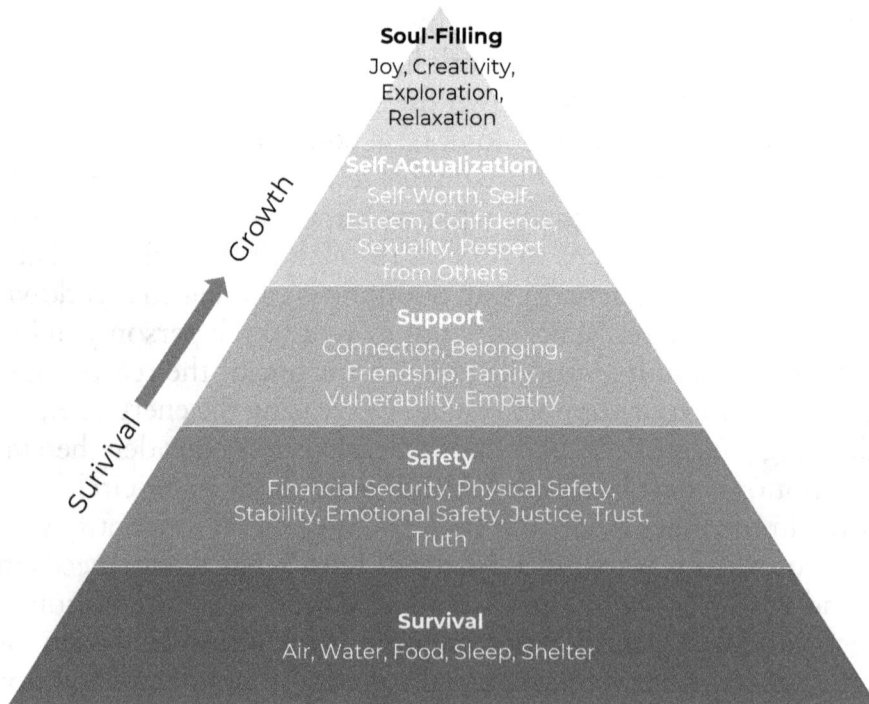

Figure 1.3 Hierarchy of Needs Chart

Use the exercise below to practice learning to see and process through your trauma responses by completing the worksheet (Figure 1.4). You can use this worksheet to process through trauma responses in the future as well.

Exercise 1–5:

1. Using the worksheet in Figure 1.4, think of a situation that was triggering for you. Which category of trauma applies to that situation? Check the boxes on the left side of the worksheet under "trauma" that apply to this situation (it may be more than one).
2. Which survival response did you react with? Check the box that applies.
3. Which safe-harboring response did you get stuck in as you tried to create safety?
4. What was the temporary benefit of that response (how did it work short-term)?
5. How did it affect you and your connection to others long-term (long-term consequences)?

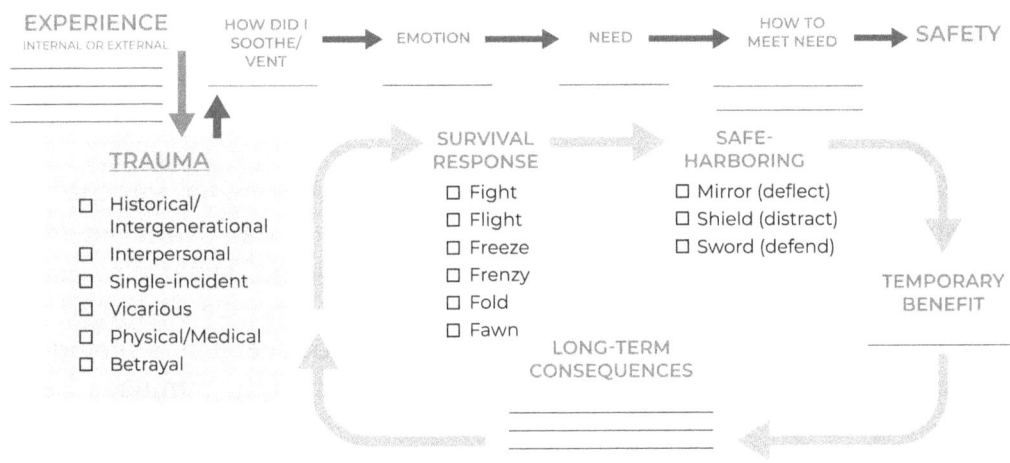

Figure 1.4 My Trauma Cycle Worksheet

The Escape Cycle

Everyone has times when we engage in some type of escape behavior, but not everyone has escape cycles. Escape cycles happen when we give up on trying to create safety and numb the pain instead of dealing with it. Escape cycles can escalate into compulsive or out-of-control patterns, but they don't start that way. Escape behaviors start with occasional use of the behavior or substance, can move to abuse of it, then can escalate to compulsive use, and become out-of-control when they escalate to the point that we can't stop them without help.

The trauma cycle gives us a reference to understand the escape cycle better. They aren't the same, but they have similarities. If you look at the diagram of the escape cycle (Figure 1.5 in section "Your Escape Cycle"), you'll see that it looks very similar to the trauma cycle. Trauma cycles are attempts to create safety. Escape cycles develop when we give up on trying to create safety and instead try to numb or escape the pain. Escape patterns numb us. We don't feel the pain anymore – we don't feel anything anymore. Behaviors that are part of the escape cycle work short-term. If you drink enough alcohol, you get drunk. If you use enough heroin, you get high. While you are high, you don't hurt.

Escape cycles escalate. We don't spin, we spiral. We get used to the behaviors and they stop working as well, so we have to escalate the behaviors in order to get the same results. Many of us have had an injury or some type of surgery and were given pain pills during our recovery. The first time we took them, they probably had a fairly strong effect. If we continue to take them, each dose has a less obvious effect. The same is true with escape patterns. For example, if you watch porn to escape or numb, rather than to connect to yourself, you'll have to watch more and more, or watch it in a riskier way, or watch more extreme material, in order to get the same escape.

Just like trauma cycles, escape cycles start with pain. At some point, the pain gets to be too much. This triggers a trauma response in us. Trauma responses are attempts to create safety. Trauma cycles turn into escape cycles when we stop trying to create safety and start trying to numb the pain instead. We give up on ourselves and/or others.

We shift into these cycles at different levels. If we think of recovery as climbing a hill, those levels can be described as trips, skirting (walking the edge of the cliff), or leaping off the cliff. We might just trip, almost like our foot slips as we're climbing up a hill. We might walk along the edge, skirting it, hoping to get the feeling of escape without falling off the cliff. Or we might leap off the cliff, jumping back into our escape patterns.

There are two different types of escape behaviors: substance behaviors and process behaviors. Substance escape behaviors are when we take chemicals from outside our body and put them into our body. These include alcohol, drugs, and sugar. Process escape behaviors are when we participate in behaviors in a way that produce chemicals in our body at much higher levels than normal human interactions produce. These include unhealthy patterns related to sex/romance, eating/food, gambling, shopping, gaming, adrenaline, and workaholism.

It's important to note that all of us have things we do to escape or get a break. Escapes are necessary as life gets overwhelming sometimes. Healthy escapes give us a break, without compromising our values. They don't set us up for situations that will cause us pain. They aren't used as a repetitive pattern to numb emotion. They don't involve escalation. We can stop them if needed. Note that what may be a healthy escape for one person might be an escape behavior for another person. For example, some people can have a couple of drinks, and it can be relaxing and help give them a break. Others may not be able to stop at a couple of drinks or may participate in behaviors that are dangerous when they drink, like not being able to tell when they aren't sober enough to drive.

When the high we get from escape behaviors wears off, we often experience shame around what we've done, and we can feel powerless around stopping the cycle. That message causes additional pain, which helps keep us trapped in the escape cycle.

Your Escape Cycle

Think of a time when you shifted into numbing your pain and utilized an escape cycle. Look for escalating (keep getting more extreme) patterns, repeated failed attempts to stop, and negative consequences from those behaviors for yourself and others. As we've talked about several times, there isn't a single substance or behavior that is an inherently unhealthy escape, so don't assume it's an escape because of what you did, think about things that make you numb. Use the worksheet in Figure 1.5 to outline your escape patterns.

Exercise 1–6:

1. What happened that was painful for you? Write your answer under "Experience" on the "My Escape Cycle" worksheet (Figure 1.5).
2. What type of trauma/pain was it? Check the appropriate box.
3. What escape response happened? Was it a slip? Were you skirting the edge? Did you panic and leap?
4. What escape behavior did you use?
5. What was the short-term benefit from using that behavior?
6. What shame messages came into your heart and mind after the high wore off?
7. What was the long-term cost of the behavior?

Similarities and Differences Between the Trauma and Escape Cycles

It's important to understand both the similarities and differences between the trauma cycle and the escape cycle. Similarities help create a context that allows us (whether you are healing from escape patterns or connected to someone who has betrayed you with their escape patterns) to better understand the how and why behind escape cycles and allows us to see them more clearly so that we have a greater ability to address them. Greater understanding helps give us more control over changing those cycles. It also helps those being hurt

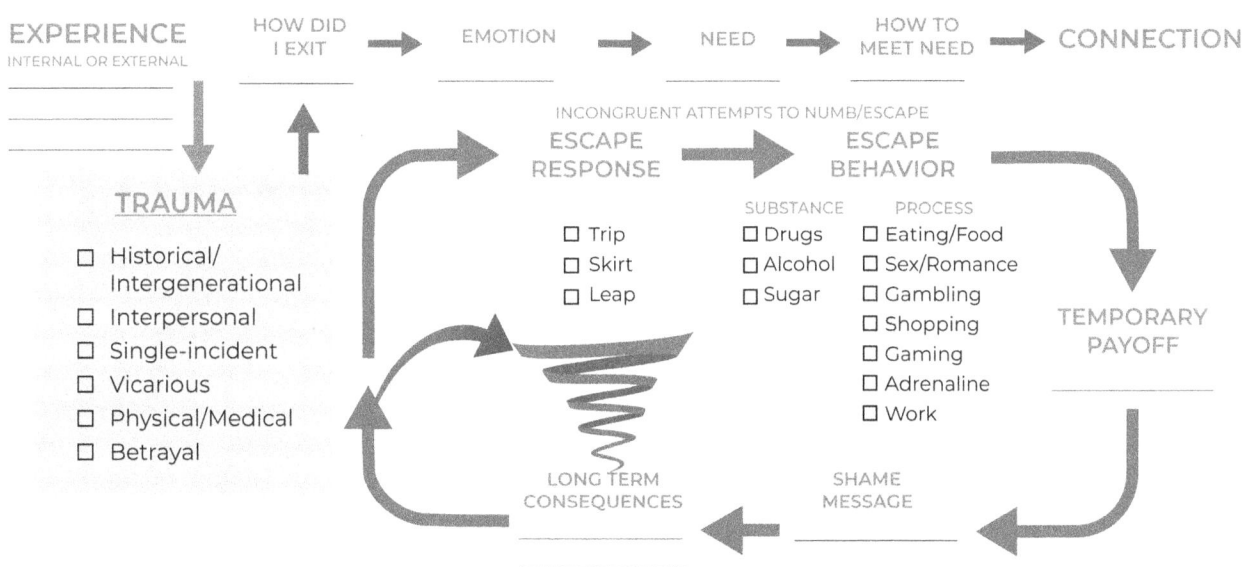

Figure 1.5 My Escape Cycle Worksheet

by the escape cycles of another to have an increased ability to create safety for themselves around the other person's escape cycles and see when changes are made to those patterns. Differences help ensure the pain experienced by the person who has been betrayed isn't minimized and they aren't held responsible for the behaviors of someone else. Differences also help those with escape patterns understand the line that is crossed when they make the shift into escape cycles.

Trauma Loop and Escape Spiral

To better understand trauma cycles and escape cycles and the connection between the two, let's look at them in a different format. Figure 1.6 shows what is called the trauma loop. The steps are the same as the bottom circle of arrows on the trauma cycle diagram, except I combined "experience" and "trauma" into "trigger." A trigger is an emotional response that carries additional weight because of similar past experiences. It's like a chain. The current experience is one link. An additional link was added every time you experienced something like that and weren't able to resolve it or create safety around it. Instead of just feeling the emotions from that experience, that link is connected to all the other links and you end up having to carry the whole chain. Because our responses to situations and experiences are based on the weight of what we have to carry around them, when we are triggered, we have a stronger response that seems warranted by the situation.

We tend to get pushed into a trauma loop/cycles when we experience a trigger. Everyone has triggers. Everyone has trauma loops. Many of my clients describe trauma responses as

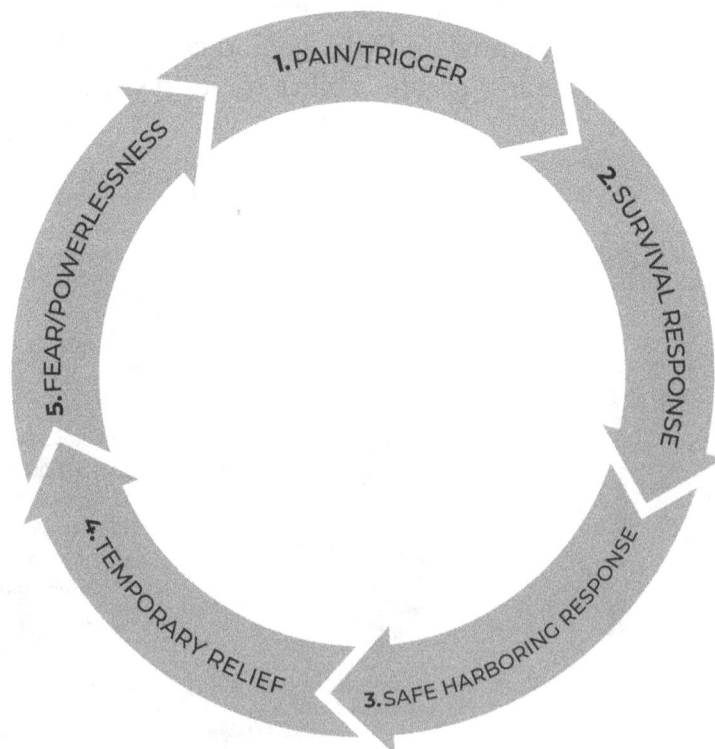

Figure 1.6 The Trauma Loop

"spinning." They feel like they are going around in a circle and can't get out of it. When we see our trauma loops and understand where they come from, we can work toward increasing our ability to stop the spinning and create safety for ourselves, as we talked about in the section about the trauma cycle.

Putting the trauma cycle in this format allows us to see the connection between the trauma cycle and the escape cycle. It also allows us to see one of the main differences. As we talked

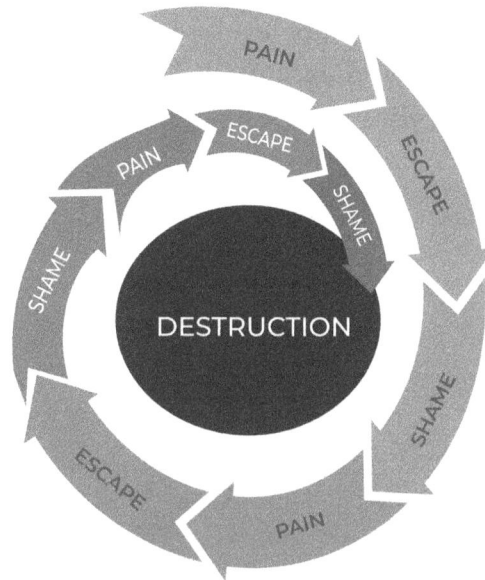

Figure 1.7 The Escape Spiral

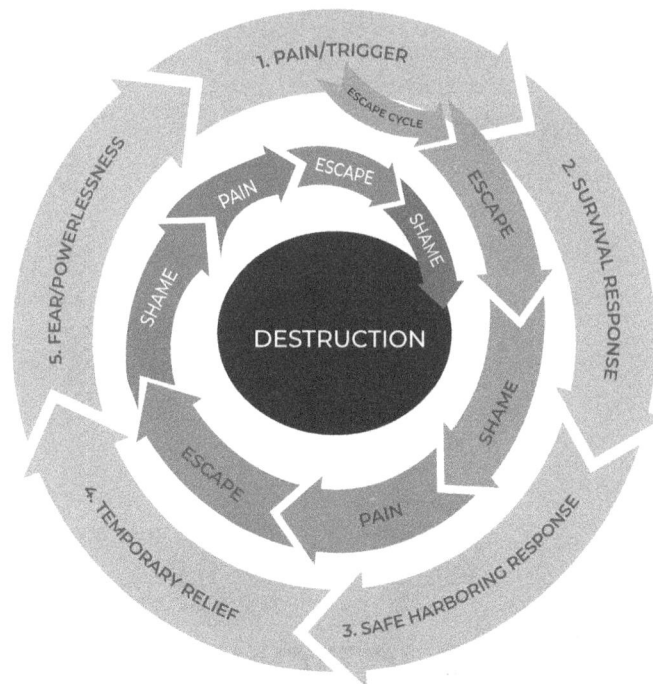

Figure 1.8 Connection Between the Trauma Loop and Escape Spiral from the Top

about earlier, while the trauma cycle spins us, escape cycles are more of a spiral. The escalation of the behaviors in order to get the same high means we don't just spin; we spiral down and eventually destroy connection to ourselves and others. Look at the diagram of the escape spiral (Figure 1.7). The escape spiral starts when we switch into escaping or numbing our pain instead of trying to create safety. The escape behavior gets us high, meaning we don't feel the pain. Then it wears off and we feel shame and powerlessness, along with the pain we tried to numb. That makes us want to escape again, starting the cycle over.

We briefly mentioned earlier that escape cycles start as trauma cycles. You can see the connection between the two in the diagrams in Figures 1.8 and 1.9. The first diagram shows the connection from the top; the second shows the connection from the side.

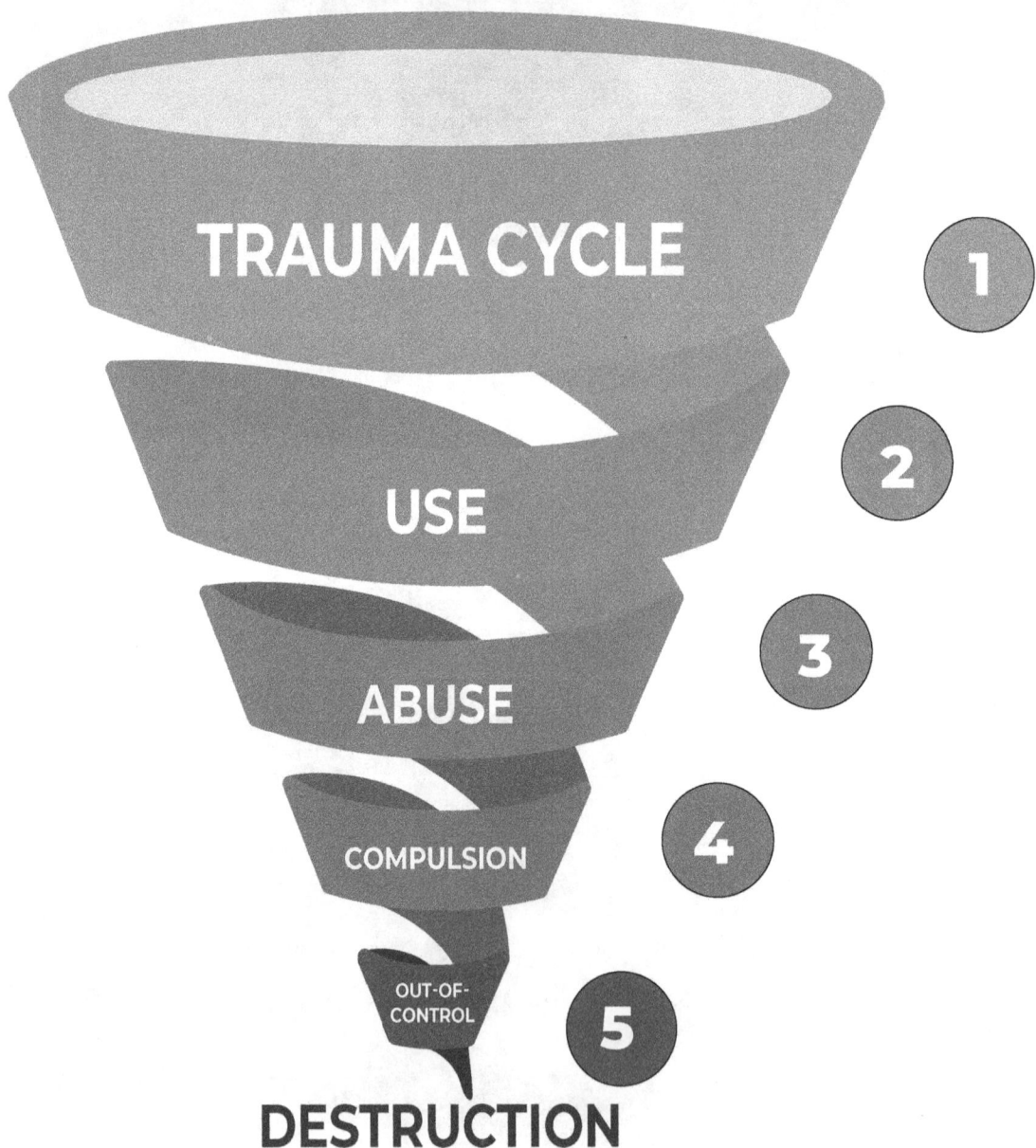

Figure 1.9 Connection Between the Trauma Loop and Escape Spiral from the Side

Exercise 1–7:

1. Can you identify a situation or experience that has triggered a strong emotional response for you?
2. Have you ever reacted to a situation and later realized your response was influenced by past unresolved experiences? What past experiences might have added "links" to that chain?
3. Now that you understand how trauma cycles and escape cycles are connected, what is one small step you could take to start breaking out of the cycle and creating real safety for yourself?

Exiting Escape Cycles

The steps to exit escape cycles are similar to the steps to exit trauma cycles. The primary difference is the first step. Rather than venting or soothing, the focus is pulling yourself away from the escape because escape cycles pull us in like a tractor beam. Come up with something to do physically and practice it over and over in your head until it's an automatic response you can activate. Your current automatic response isn't helpful (although it may have been in the past), so you have to retrain your brain. This is similar to knowing how to respond if you catch on fire. Each of us knows "stop, drop, and roll." We had to memorize those steps because our automatic response is to run. It's one of the few survival responses that make the situation worse. To break out of your escape cycle, distract yourself. Yodel, talk in an accent, jump up and run out of the room, start singing, do jumping jacks. Whatever fits best for you.

Once you've exited your automatic pattern, use the same tools we discussed earlier in relation to exiting the trauma cycle. Identify your emotions, use those to figure out what your needs are, and then consider solutions that will meet your needs in healthy ways.

Exercise 1–8:

1. How do you know that you're trapped in your escape cycle?
2. What can you do to distract yourself when you are stuck in your escape cycle?

Super Short Summary:

Early recovery (Phase 1) focuses on creating emotional safety through truth. The education component of early recovery focuses on trauma and escape cycles. When working to connect to yourself and others, abuse, deception, or escape patterns must be tackled first to create safety for each individual involved. Trauma cycles are responses to unresolved pain. Escape cycles start with trauma cycles, but escalate into escapes when we try to numb the pain rather than address the situation.

Chapter Questions:

1. What did you connect to the most in this chapter?
2. What steps are you taking to apply this material to your life?

Honesty
Disclosure/Amends and Defining Self

The honesty component of early recovery is understanding your story, how you got here, and who you would like to become. This is true whether you are struggling with problematic patterns of behaviors or healing from betrayal. If you are healing from betrayal, often many of the puzzle pieces are held by the person who has betrayed you, so in many cases, talking with that person and having them answer your questions through the therapeutic disclosure process can be an essential part as you begin to build a sense of safety again. Whether or not you go through the disclosure process, sorting through your story and deciding where you want to go from here is essential.

Therapeutic Disclosure

The disclosure process looks different for each person and each relationship. In some cases, you may already have explored what happened at the level you and anyone you are in a relationship with need. In other cases, exploring it at a deeper level is helpful. In general, the disclosure process resolves questions about violations of a relational contract. If all of your questions have been answered, whether they are questions about what you did and how you got to a place that you did it, or questions about what your significant other did and how they got to a place that they did those things, you may not need to do additional work around sorting through the situation. If you or those connected to you still have questions, some level of therapeutic disclosure might be helpful.

Drs. John and Julie Gottman, who founded the Gottman Institute and have specialized in working with relationships for the last 50 years, discuss the importance of processing through questions following betrayal. They state that relationships will stay stuck unless the questions are processed. This is explained by a theory called the Zeigarnik Effect, which is almost a hundred years old. It was first discovered by Bluma Zeigarnik, a Soviet researcher in Berlin in the 1920s. She watched waiters take orders without writing anything down, When she talked to the waiters after the bills were paid, they no longer remembered what the orders were. Her studies showed that we spend a lot of our mental bandwidth focusing on unresolved issues.

While Zeigarnik's studies were done a century ago, the ideas behind those studies are the foundational concepts behind current trauma treatments such as eye movement

DOI: 10.4324/9781003623359-4

desensitization and reprocessing (EMDR) and somatic experiencing (Fox, 2020; Riordan, 2022). Our brains get stuck trying to make sense of things that happen to us until we process through them. This is directly tied to the trauma cycle we discussed in Chapter 1.

The process of looking at what happened can also be very helpful for those struggling with problematic behaviors. Many clients I've worked with say that they didn't understand their own story until they put it together in their disclosure process. Whether you are struggling with problematic patterns or healing from betrayal, and whether you are in a relationship or not, I recommend sorting through what happened in a way that is therapeutic for you. This will be different for each person and each relationship.

There is currently very little research on whether or not disclosure is helpful following betrayal. A study published in 2023 (Stavrova et al.) found that keeping infidelity a secret is more damaging to relationships and to individuals who have betrayed. Another study on the topic involved reviewing material from a previous study, which followed couples who attended couples counseling sessions over a period of five years. After the study (Marín et al., 2014) was completed, another group (Barraca & Polanski, 2021) reviewed the material and found that the questionnaires revealed some information about disclosing betrayal. There were 134 couples in the study. Among those with no betrayal, 77% of them (88 out of 115) were still together after five years. Fourteen of the couples indicated there was disclosed betrayal, and 57% of them were still together at the end of the study. There was undisclosed betrayal for five of the couples and only one of those relationships, 20% of the couples in that category, was still intact at the end of the study.

One of the most common concerns around going through the disclosure process is if it's really worth digging all that up again. I often hear "Shouldn't we just move forward? That feels like we're going backwards." Dr. Janice Caudill, one of the authors of the Full Disclosure books, uses a story from Egyptian mythology to illustrate the need for the disclosure process. She tells the story of Isis and Osiris, a husband and wife who were deeply in love. Their brother (yes, they were siblings, it's mythology), Seth, was jealous and killed Osiris. After Osiris was dead, Seth tore his body into pieces, hiding it all over the world. As Isis grieved, she searched the world for each piece of the man she loved. She found them all and brought them together again, "re-membering" him (one word for body parts is "members"), making him whole, and breathing life back into him. This is a very brief summary of the story, but this illustrates the role of disclosure in the healing process. We are re-membering what happened and, in the process, taking steps to help make you whole again. It is very difficult to move forward in a relationship without knowing what happened, having the appropriate person take accountability for it, and taking the steps to repair it. It is possible to heal even if the person who betrayed you is not willing to go through a disclosure process at the level needed for your relationship. You will need to sort through the steps that are right for you moving forward and determine the boundaries you need to set to create safety for yourself and your relationship, if it continues.

As I stated earlier, the disclosure process looks different for each individual and each relationship. The Connected Recovery® Disclosure books can help you walk through the process and determine the best way for you to navigate this part of healing. I highly recommend you not go through this process on your own. Find therapists who are familiar with treating infidelity and betrayal and are familiar with disclosures to help you sort through understanding your experience, what to share about your experience within your relationship, and how to share it. Changing the patterns and processing through truth will be painful. It can also be incredibly healing. If you try to do the process on your own, the chances of the material being processed, accurate, and complete are very low. Trying to do this process on your own or with therapists who are not familiar with the disclosure process will likely make the situation worse rather than promote healing. I also highly recommend you work with clinicians who approach the process as part of healing rather than as punishment.

There are situations where going through a therapeutic disclosure is not helpful and may even make the situation worse. Sometimes the person or people who have been betrayed don't have unanswered questions and already have all the information they need. If you are involved in any type of lawsuit or if you are going through a divorce, it may be unwise, emotionally and/or legally, to go through this process until the lawsuit is resolved or the divorce is finalized. Talk to your lawyer and figure out what is best for you. If one or more members of a relationship refuse to attend therapy or get therapeutic support, disclosure may not be helpful or safe. In general, if someone's reactions make sharing or discussing information unsafe, then disclosure shouldn't be done. Finally, if there are major life events or health issues, such as death of a loved one, cancer, or high-risk pregnancy, disclosure may be more harmful than helpful. Talk with your clinician about how to navigate your specific situation.

Exercise 2–1:

1. What are your thoughts about therapeutic disclosure?
2. Talk to your therapist and/or group about how you would like to move forward with this step of the process. If you are going through this process in a primary relationship, make sure each of you has a separate therapist familiar with the process to support you through it.
3. If you have gone through an informal disclosure or a disclosure that was unhelpful for you, process that with your therapist and/or group (I realize that one question in this book will not provide the support necessary to process through this – I wanted to highlight it to ensure that it was addressed).

Stages of Grief

Seeing the ways we have betrayed ourselves and potentially others or finding out how we were betrayed often leads us to the stages of grief. The traditional model of the stages of grief developed by Elisabeth Kübler-Ross (1969) includes five stages: denial, anger, depression, bargaining, and acceptance. I've changed a few of the names and added a stage because it was missing from the original model.

Shock

I've renamed the first stage of grief "shock" rather than "denial." Denial sends the message that we are deliberately refusing to look at something. The first stage of grief is not being in denial. It's closer to physical shock. If we're in a serious accident and our body is very damaged, we can go into shock. Our heart rate slows, our breathing slows, our blood pressure drops, and our brain shifts into much lower functioning. All of these responses help us to survive using less of the resources we need to live. This happens to give us a better chance of living through the situation.

The first stage of grief is the emotional version of physical shock. It's our mind and heart filtering the pain so we survive the situation. If we felt the whole weight of the pain at once, we might not be able to live through it. Every stage of grief has a purpose. This stage gives us glimpses into the pain so we can process through it a chunk at a time. In this stage of grief, we can't believe the situation is real. We think, and might even say out loud, "this can't be happening" or "this can't be my life." Don't try to force yourself out of this stage. It wears off as you live through the experience. We'll talk about empathy for self in detail in Chapter 9 of this book, but for now, give yourself grace. Understand that it makes sense you're feeling shock. Again, it's not about being in denial. You aren't just refusing to look at it.

As we talk through these stages, realize that we don't go through them in order. It's not a linear process. At the beginning, we feel a whole lot of shock and very little acceptance. At the end, we feel a whole lot of acceptance and very little shock. The rest is a mess of all six, depending on the day, hour, or possibly minute. Even when you move into strong acceptance, you can still have other stages show up occasionally.

Anger

The second stage of grief is anger. Anger is the energy behind the pain. It tells us that something is wrong and someone, either ourselves or others or both, is being hurt. This energy gives us the power to move forward. The anger we feel might be pointed at others, ourselves, or even God or the universe. "How could you?!?!?" is very often connected to this stage. Let yourself feel the anger. Even if the anger is at God. An all-powerful being who sees into your heart can handle your true emotions. It's ok to be mad at God.

Find ways to let it out that are safe for you and others. Often this includes physical activity. Go to a rage room or somewhere that offers axe-throwing. Buy a bag of ice and break it up with a hammer. Pick one that looks like it's melted and refrozen so it's more solid. I'd recommend either taking it out of the plastic bag first or putting it in a pillowcase so it's easier to clean up. You'll destroy the pillowcase in this activity, so use an old one or buy one from a second-hand store. If you express anger better in writing, then write. If you prefer creating art to express emotions, paint or sculpt or collage. Listening to music that expresses a similar level of anger might be helpful as well.

Raw Emotions

The third stage of grief was originally called "depression," but it's more than that. It's the raw emotions connected to the grief. It's the pain. This can include depression. We might not be able to even get out of bed, or might feel like we're living in a fog. It also can include anguish and despair, which feel sharper to me than depression. We might not even have words for this stage. It might be ending up curled up on the floor, sobbing.

When you are in this stage of grief, let yourself feel. Like the anger stage of grief, sometimes it can be helpful to express it. Sob or scream if you need to. Write the pain down in journaling or poetry if you process through writing. Use art if you process that way. Music has a lot of emotion connected to it, so listening to music that expresses emotions similar to what you're feeling can be helpful as well. We're going to talk about shame in the next section, but don't shame yourself for the emotions you feel. Emotions aren't bad or good. They just give us information. We'll talk about this in detail in Chapter 6. In this case, the emotions are showing you how deeply you were impacted by what happened.

Bargaining

The fourth stage of grief is bargaining. Bargaining is "how could I change the story so it has a different ending." We wonder what we could have done differently in the past, or what someone else could have done differently. Maybe if we hadn't met someone. Maybe if it had come to light sooner. Maybe if we had handled a situation differently. Maybe if we'd said something or not said something. "If only…" This stage of grief also tries to come up with solutions that will fix the situation moving forward. "What if…" What if we do or say it this way.

This stage of grief helps us figure out what to do as we move forward. In my experience, this is the stage of grief we are most likely to get stuck in, although that can happen with any stage. If you get stuck in any specific stage or in the grief process in general, get help. Give yourself time and space to wish things had happened differently. In general, the first year is the hardest. That doesn't mean that all your pain disappears the second year or the third, but as you process through it and as you move forward, the pain will get better. It will decrease in either intensity or frequency or both. Keep processing the information, considering what you have the ability to change moving forward.

Making Meaning

The fifth stage of grief is the one I added. I call it "making meaning." This is the redemptive part of grief. It helps you take back your power. This stage of grief focuses on the good you choose to do with what you went through. I don't mean that anything that was done to you that hurt you was good. When we go through painful experiences and process through them, we take the pain we went through and decide how it will change us and change the way we interact with others.

The quote "I am not what happened to me. I am what I choose to become" is attributed to Carl Jung. He never actually said that, but it explains this stage of grief. We may not have had any ability to control what happened to us, what others did to us, but we can choose what we want to do with it and the way it impacted us. We can choose what we want to become. What are you going to decide to do with what has happened to you? What do you want to learn from this? Considering those questions doesn't mean you're ok with someone else hurting you or you are ok with the things you've done if you're processing through ways you betrayed yourself and others. You're in the situation. What do you want to make of what you've gone through?

I've had clients who recognized that they developed more empathy for themselves and others. I've had others who appreciated the tools they learned and that they chose to use the situation to process through experiences, patterns, and behaviors and become more connected to themselves. Maybe you decide to use what you've gone through to write a book or help others who are dealing with pain similar to what you experienced.

Acceptance

The final stage of grief is acceptance. This doesn't mean you're ok with what happened. I love Michael J. Fox's definition of acceptance (2012). He said, "Acceptance doesn't mean resignation; it means understanding that something is what it is and that there's got to be a way through it." Acceptance allows us to move forward and to work toward feeling peace. Peace doesn't mean what happened was a good thing. It doesn't mean you don't need to take steps to prevent the same thing from happening again. It's actually just the opposite. We can't feel peace if we aren't safe. We can't be safe if we don't set up boundaries so we won't be hurt in the same way in the future.

Exercise 2–2:

1. Does this align with what you've experienced when you've gone through grief in your life?
2. Are you currently grieving something? If so, which stages have you recently experienced?

Defining Self

As I stated earlier, recovery is the process of recovering yourself, figuring out who you are and who you want to become. While the work we've explored thus far will help with that, at this point in the process, it's helpful to pause and define this specifically. If you have gone through the disclosure process, you may find it helpful to refer to the work you did as you create the lists in Exercise 2–3 below.

Many of those who have gone through the 12 steps have done some work in this area, as step four of the 12 steps is to "make a searching and fearless moral inventory" (Alcoholics Anonymous World Services, 2001) of ourselves. The approach outlined below is a bit different as the AA 12 steps focuses only on our resentments, fears, guilt, and shame. We also need to consider our strengths, accomplishments, abilities, and potential. We are not just defined by our failings. We must look clearly at the parts of ourselves we don't like in order to fully accept ourselves and embrace who we are, but a complete picture of ourselves includes much more than just the aspects we struggle with. Also, it's important to recognize that "fearless" does not mean it isn't scary to create these lists; it means we don't let our fears stop us.

Exercise 2–3:

1. What thoughts come to mind as you prepare to take the steps to look at yourself more clearly?
2. What are you most afraid of?
3. What are you most excited about?

Resentments

We're going to start with resentments. Like all emotions, resentment isn't bad or good, it gives us information. It lets us know that we are giving more of ourselves, or more is being taken from us, than we are getting back. It highlights a deficit in the process. It's important to recognize that deficits are not necessarily anyone's fault. They might indicate boundaries or patterns, either of which may be related to our own behaviors and/or the behavior of others we need to change. The point of this part of the process isn't to blame others or shame yourself. You probably will have realizations that highlight changes you need to make regarding what others are able to take from you and what you give to others, but the point of this isn't to beat yourself or anyone else up. It's to identify the areas of your life that need to be changed so you can be whole.

Additionally, when you consider resentments, explore how your resentments are impacting you. This might indicate ways resentments are protecting you, or it might indicate behaviors or thoughts that don't align with who you are or who you want to be. A colleague of mine, Dr. James Taylor, asks his clients "What does it buy you and what does it cost you?" Everything we do makes sense in context, meaning there's a reason we do it. If we examine it, we can figure out if the way we are handling the situation is the best fit for what we need to be safe and who we want to be.

Exercise 2–4:

1. Pause your reading and make a list of everyone and everything you resent and what you resent them for. This likely includes more than just people in your life. It may include institutions or organizations, ideas or beliefs, situations and experiences. Resentment can manifest as anger or bitterness against someone or something. It can be seen as times you were wronged or things that were done against you. It can also be things that were done that hurt you, even if they weren't done specifically against you. As with any work you do in this process, create a situation in which it's safe to write in an unfiltered format. Password protect the document on your computer or buy a safe to keep your notebooks in if you prefer to write it down instead of type it. Save it somewhere where others cannot access it. (Note that you will probably not be able to create a complete list the first time you work on it. Use a format that you can come back and add to as you remember or realize things.)

2. Review your list and consider how each resentment is benefiting you and then what each one is costing you as well. Add that information to your list.
3. Review your list and consider if the current way you are handling each situation is the best fit for you or if there are different boundaries and approaches that might work better. Sometimes this work helps us to see pain that needs to be processed. If that is the case, talk to your therapist about how best to process that pain so you don't have to carry it with you anymore.

Fears

Having created your list of resentments, let's move onto fears. This is somewhat similar to the process we just used to create a resentments list, except in this case we're looking at what or who you are afraid of. Those fears may be historical (meaning they were created a long time ago, but we haven't processed through them completely yet), or they may be current. It can feel uncomfortable to consider our fears because fear can indicate vulnerability. This step can be especially difficult if you weren't emotionally safe in some major relationship/connection in your life, such as in the family you grew up in or a current or previous primary relationship. If that's the case, or if this step is difficult for you, process those emotions with your therapist and/or group.

There may also be shame connected to feeling fear. We may have been taught that if we feel afraid, we're weak or cowardly. We'll talk more about shame in just a bit, but just as we've discussed earlier, emotions, including fear, aren't bad or good, they just give us information. Just like any other emotion, fear gives us information that allows us to identify our needs so they can be met. Courage isn't the absence of fear, it's taking the steps we need to take even when we feel fear. It's acknowledging our fears and working through them. In her TED talk, *The Power of Vulnerability*, Brown (2010) defines courage as telling "the story of who you are with your whole heart." Our whole heart encompasses all our emotions, including fear.

As you sort through your fears, your resentments list may be helpful to refer to as resentments are often fueled by fear. As with the resentments list, realize that as you go through the process of recovering from the pain that caused you to read this book, you will likely see additional fears that you didn't recognize earlier. This is a living document, meaning you can add to it as you learn more about yourself. Use a format that allows you to do so. Also, as with the other steps we've talked about, take the steps to protect this document so that you feel safe to be completely honest as you create it.

Exercise 2–5:

1. Start by considering what's coming up for you as you consider listing your fears. Process through any concerns or triggers you have with your therapist and/or group.

2. Make a list of your fears. What or who are you afraid of? This could include individuals, events, emotions, or organizations. Why?
3. Consider your list of resentments. What are the underlying fears connected to each item on your list? Why do you resent the individuals, organizations, or events? What are you afraid will happen, is happening, or has already happened?

Deception

I don't love the word "deception" because it often has a lot of shame connected to it, but I've found using that word helps people see themselves and what they've gone through more clearly. Where there is long lasting pain, whether that pain is from childhood or adulthood, often there is deception, because deception can prevent us from seeing a situation and taking steps to protect ourselves and heal from what happened. Merriam-Webster (n.d.-d) defines deception as "the act of causing someone to accept as true or valid what is false or invalid." This can show up due to lack of awareness within ourselves or others, deep-seated fears that lead to denial in us or others, or facades created by us or others. Deception is often unconscious. It might be continuing to believe something taught, like family roles and rules, which we'll talk about later in this book, or organizational beliefs taught by subcultures we are part of, because we haven't thought to question it. In order to heal as completely as possible, we need to examine our lives and see who we are and what we've gone through as clearly as possible.

Deception is often used to try to protect ourselves, or used by others to try and prevent pain for them. It actually doesn't protect; it traps us because we don't have the information to make an informed decision about the situation. Because of this, it's important to consider the role deception plays in our lives. As we go through this step, consider how you might have deceived others or yourself and how others might have deceived you.

It can also be painful to consider how others deceived us. It can seem like we aren't being fair to them and aren't considering the whole picture or aren't taking responsibility for our part. Just as with the other parts of this process, the point of this isn't to shame you or blame others; it's to free you and help you process through the pain you've experienced.

Exercise 2–6:

1. Consider the experiences you have gone through. Where might deception (by you or others) have played a role?
2. What did you see about yourself that was helpful?
3. What did you see about yourself that was painful (this may include parts of your answer to the previous questions)?
4. How did it influence your view of yourself?

Shame

Very often as we explore resentments, fears, and deception, shame comes up as we're highlighting the painful and unhealthy patterns we've had in our lives. Note that shame is different than feeling ashamed. Feeling ashamed means you made a mistake or did something incongruent with who you are, and you feel badly about it. Shame is grounded in the belief that we either have to be perfect or we suck as human beings. Shame attaches itself to emotions and tells us that our mistake or mistakes define us and are irreparable. Let's explore what shame is, where it comes from, and how to deal with it.

Often identifying and considering our faulty core beliefs can be helpful in exploring shame. Faulty core beliefs are lies about ourselves or how others connect to us that we've been taught (as in we learned them from other people in our lives) or developed as a result of trauma or dysfunction (disconnection). They feel very real. In some cases, parts of some of them may have been accurate at certain points of our lives or in certain connections/relationships.

In his book *Facing the Shadow*, Dr. Patrick Carnes (2001) created a list of faulty core beliefs that often come from escape patterns. Each is shame-based, meaning that they feel unfixable. As part of a conversation I had with Dr. Barbara Steffens and Dr. Jill Manning (personal communication, 2019), they created a list of faulty core beliefs that often come from being betrayed. These are shame-based as well. I've found that my clients often connect to faulty core beliefs from both lists, regardless of their personal history.

It's important to recognize that while it's common to struggle with these core beliefs, not everyone struggling with problematic patterns of behavior or healing from betrayal connects to each of them, or possibly any of them. If you read through these and they don't connect to you, don't try to force yourself to fit them into your experience. As with every other tool or idea in these books, there will be some that fit very well and others that don't fit at all. Try them on for size, sort of like an outfit. Keep the parts that fit and leave the rest. You are unique and your story is unique. One part of recovering yourself is learning to step out of automatically accepting boxes other people try to put you in. You cannot heal by pretending to be someone you aren't.

Also keep in mind that you may not connect to these now but may go over the list again in the future and find that you connect to items on one or both lists at that point. That just means you're processing at a different level and have had new realizations about yourself.

The four faulty core beliefs listed by Dr. Patrick Carnes (2001) are:

1. I am basically a bad, unworthy person.
2. No one will love me as I am.
3. My needs will never be met if I rely on others to meet them.
4. Escape (Dr. Carnes said "sex," but we're replacing that with "escape" in connection to the escape cycle) is my most important need.

The list of faulty core beliefs potentially originating from experiencing betrayal that Dr. Barbara Steffens and Dr. Jill Manning (personal communication, 2019) compiled include:

1. I am now unlovable.
2. I am broken beyond repair.

3. If I was enough, I would not have been betrayed.
4. I can never trust anyone.
5. I am either too much or not enough.
6. I cannot trust myself.

In order to see ourselves clearly, both our strengths and our weaknesses, we need to separate the voices of others that have taught us that we aren't worthy of love or connection. Why would you want to connect to yourself if you believe you are inherently unworthy or unlovable? Why would you want to connect to others if you believe no one will love you or meet your needs, or that you can never trust anyone, or you are too much or not enough? How could you stand to process your struggles if you believe they are unfixable and define who you are at your core? And how could you trust connection to others if you believe you will be rejected and alone if they see who you really are? These core beliefs hold us hostage from connection to ourselves and connection to others. They stop us from being able to see ourselves clearly, to claim our strengths, and see our weaknesses.

Exercise 2–7:

1. Take the time to go through the lists above, determine which faulty core beliefs resonate with you, and process through those with your therapist and/or group.
2. Rewrite those beliefs from the list so that the shame is removed from them, so they are accurate and balanced. For example, "I am either too much or not enough" might be rewritten as something like "I have strong emotions and a lot of deep wounds from things I've experienced. I don't know how to trust connection. There will be times when my emotions feel overwhelming, and times when I need help, but that is part of being human. I have people who love me and have fought for connection with me, and I am learning to love myself."

Now that we've taken the time to understand a little bit more about shame, let's work on processing through it more completely. The Processing Shame Worksheet (available at ConnectedRecoveryTraining.com) walks you through that. I'll include an example in the following paragraphs so you can see it illustrated, then we'll take the time to have you fill one out on your own. You can use this worksheet for relapses into escape behaviors or relational patterns, or even just to process day-to-day struggles that include shame. Note that shame is usually connected to deep emotions and experiences, so the processing that comes up as you explore this is often complex.

Here's an example of a day-to-day issue.

Let's say you make a mistake at work. You forget to respond to an email. In this case, it's not a hugely important email that would make or break your job, just one that you "should" have responded to. I put "should" in quotation marks as should often indicates the added weight of shame.

The emotions you might be feeling may be inadequate and guilty. The underlying needs might be confidence and respect of others. You can meet those needs in healthy ways by apologizing for not responding to the email and figuring out what happened that caused you to miss responding to it.

Now let's dig into the shame related to it. What did you think about yourself when you figured out that you didn't respond to the email? Maybe "I suck" or "Man, I am so incompetent!" Both of those have weight that goes beyond missing responding to an email. The message connected to those phrases might be "If I make a mistake at work, I'm a screw up."

Where might you have learned that message? Maybe you heard your mom or dad say it about themselves. Maybe you were taught that straight A's were the only acceptable grade. The first message would have been from your parents. The second might have been your parents or family members, your teachers, or you may have made it up yourself.

Let's focus on hearing your parents say it about themselves. They may have learned it from how they grew up. Maybe they used that to help them succeed. Shame can feel motivating, but it weighs you down just as much as it pushes you forward. They also may have not wanted you to feel the pain that comes from mistakes, so they pushed you to not make them.

The next question asks you how that message influenced your life. Maybe it pushed you to not make as many mistakes. Or it could have done the opposite and made you believe that since you couldn't be perfect, it wasn't worth trying. Maybe you've carried the weight of your mistakes, no matter how big they are, with you. If so, you aren't the only one! At least once a week I see some meme or quote on social media that says something about remembering every mistake they've ever made and replaying them in their heads, or about mistakes we make being carved in stone for us while mistakes others make are more like writing it in the sand. However it influenced you, it likely increased the emotional weight you've had to carry every day.

Now let's consider if there are any parts of this message that would be helpful to keep. Remember, we're taking the shame off of the message. A more balanced version of this message might be that you consider it respectful and helpful to respond to work emails in a timely fashion and that working to figure out how to do that on a more regular basis would be helpful.

Finally, having processed the shame, let's rewrite the message. In this case, it might end up being something like "When I make a mistake, it adds to the work I have to do, so I'd rather not make them. I recognize that I'm human though, and mistakes will happen. When I make a mistake, rather than beat myself up, I'll use it to evaluate how I'm doing things and what might be out of balance, or if there are tools that might be helpful for me to add."

As you start using this worksheet to process through shame, you'll likely start seeing patterns. These patterns are related to faulty core beliefs. Faulty core beliefs aren't just formed from escaping and betrayal. They come from all sorts of experiences. In the example above, the faulty core belief might be "I have to be perfect or I'm not good enough." Understanding our faulty core beliefs is the first step toward freeing us from shame and increasing peace and connection in our lives.

Exercise 2–8:

1. Consider times or situations or emotions that often or almost always produce feelings of shame in you. Pick one and complete a Processing Shame Worksheet (see ConnectedRecoveryTraining.com) around that scenario or emotion.
2. Using the lists above and the information from the worksheet, begin a list of your faulty core beliefs. As situations come up in the future that bring up shame, add to this list and process through those beliefs with your therapist.

Strengths, Accomplishments, and Abilities

We've talked about resentments, fears, and shame. Let's move on to the other side of the equation. Strengths, accomplishments, abilities, and potential are all connected to each other. Strengths are the abilities or talents that come naturally to us. Abilities are learned skills or abilities that can be cultivated over time. Accomplishments are measurable outcomes resulting from applying our strengths and abilities. Potential looks at our strengths, abilities, and accomplishments and considers our capacity for future growth, achievement, or development. The combination of all four helps us consider what we're good at, what we can learn, what we have done with both our strengths and our abilities, and what we want to do going forward.

Interestingly, the activities you've done to consider what your resentments, fears, and shame might be connected to can also be used to create a list of your strengths, accomplishments, abilities, and potential. Consider the painful experiences you've gone through. Usually when we think of the traumas we've faced, we explore the wounds they created in us. This time we're going to shift into looking at those traumas as experiences that highlight our strengths, accomplishments, and abilities, and help to identify our potential.

I want to pause here and say that pretty much every client I've ever worked with says the phrase "but it's not as bad as what others have gone through." That will always be true. You will always be able to find someone whose experience is worse than yours. This doesn't invalidate your pain or your experience. In order to process through the experiences we've gone through, we need to look at them, look at how they influenced us, and work through the messages we got from what we went through.

With that context, let's look at the experiences that created wounds (emotional, psychological, mental, and physical) in you. How did you make it through those? It takes a monumental amount of strength to make it through hell and survive. I know you probably weren't given a choice, but you still made it through. Also, often we learn the most from the pain we experience. This does not give credit to the person (or institution or experience) that hurt us; it is what we chose to do with what we went through. It's how we created redemption out of pain. It's the acceptance part of grief – it is what it is, and this is how I'm going to move forward and what I'm going to choose to do with it. Our abilities allow us to learn and apply those lessons. The choices we make throughout this process indicate our strengths, accomplishments, and abilities.

Exercise 2–9:

1. Referring to the work you've done in other exercises, consider the painful experiences you've gone through in your life. As you do that, list the tools you used to survive each experience (your **strengths**).
2. Once you've added the tools you used, consider what you learned from each one (your **accomplishments**) and add that to the list.
3. Make a third row and add what **abilities** allowed you to learn those lessons.
4. Make a list of the strengths, accomplishments, and abilities you discovered as part of this process. Look for patterns and/or connections. What do you notice?
5. How does this impact your understanding of and connection to the person who went through those experiences? What do you see that you may not have seen before? If this were someone else, what would you think or say about them? Often, it's more difficult to see or claim good things about ourselves than others.
6. Now work to realize those realizations are about you. It may be helpful to work with your therapist and/or group on this step.

Potential

Potential is what we can become. Potential is maximizing the best version of ourselves. Potential is what we choose to do with the pain we've gone through, whether it is the result of our own decisions or it is the pain caused by the choices and behaviors of others. Sometimes potential is the person we could have been if we hadn't gotten trapped in our trauma or escape cycles. Often, it's the person we choose to become despite what we've gone through, using our experiences as building blocks to help us become even more than we could have been without the pain we experienced.

This ties into the acceptance stage of grief. Acceptance isn't "I'm ok with this," it's "this is what happened, and this is how I'm going to move forward with this as part of my story." We can't change the past and, in most cases, we can't pick the cards we've been dealt. We can decide what to do with what we've gone through, what others have done to us, and/or what we've done to ourselves. This is redemption – finding peace and hope in the pain.

Please note that taking this step doesn't eliminate the need for boundaries. Quite the opposite; we can't take this step without creating and enforcing boundaries so what we become is protected from destruction. Additionally, working through your potential is not a finite step. It's a process that will continue throughout your recovery, and throughout your life. As you work through each step of this process, you will expand your potential and increase your ability to create safety for yourself and safety within your relationships. Every step we take in that direction helps us move toward our potential.

Potential is our hope for the future and the counterbalance to everything terrible you did or experienced. You realize at a soul level that the pain you've gone through can be healed. When you use that pain to help yourself and others, you become more whole. You have potential for good. For healing. Escape cycles and betrayal can be so devastating to everyone involved. Potential is the chance to change the narrative. It brings hope and healing to see what you can do with the pain you've gone through. One person who struggled with problematic patterns (anonymous, personal communication, 2022) said "You see the destruction. You see the pain. You see the weight of what you've gone through. To believe that you could use that for good, it's almost too good to be true."

The potential for good isn't limited to those with problematic patterns of behavior. Many of those who have been betrayed find a much deeper connection to themselves as they go through the process of recovering from the betrayal they've experienced. This deeper connection allows them to find joy and relate to others in a way and at a level they haven't experienced before. They learn things about themselves and connection that not only help to heal them, but those around them.

Whatever brought you here, it can be terrifying to consider your potential, because it brings hope. Hope is one of the scariest emotions we can feel, because if we feel hope, it increases our ability to feel pain and to experience loss. If we hope for nothing, we have nothing to lose. However, without hope, we have nothing. Hope starts the process of rebuilding ourselves and our lives.

Exercise 2–10:

1. Think about who and what you want to be. Make a list of goals, personality traits, and skills you would like to develop.
2. Consider the pain you've experienced and what you've learned thus far in the recovery process and throughout your life. Refer to the previous exercise (Exercise 2–9) in the "Strengths, Accomplishments, and Abilities" section. Make a list of what you want to take with you as you move forward.
3. Consider who you currently are. Create a self-portrait. Something that represents you. This could be a written list, a collage, a Pinterest board, a playlist of songs, or any other type of creation that fits for you.
4. Using the lists from Exercise 2–9, now create a portrait of who you want to be. Again, use any medium you'd like (music, pictures, words, etc.).

Personal Compass

At this point, we've done the work to see our resentments, fears, and the role deception plays in our life. We've done the work to separate the voices of shame from our core beliefs and recreate a list that does not have voices from our past defining it and keeping us hostage. We've considered our strengths, accomplishments, and abilities. We've created something that expresses our potential, who we want to be and hope we can become. Now we're ready to figure out how we might want to move forward and what will guide us in that process.

Dr. Janice Caudill, one of the founders of APSATS, has an exercise she calls "My Personal Compass" (2012), which she gave me permission to include in this book. I've found this exercise to be very helpful as a foundational tool because it helps you determine what to focus on and how to guide yourself as you move forward. As with many of the tools in these books, your compass may change over time. It's often helpful to revisit it at different stages of your recovery process. This exercise can also be redone in each phase of recovery with a different focus each time. In early recovery we focus on creating it for ourselves. In middle recovery, we create a relational version of it, either for our primary relationship or our connection to others. In late recovery, we create a version of it related to sexuality (don't let that freak you out – it will not be used to force you to do anything you don't want to do and aren't ready for).

A visual of the Personal Compass is available at ConnectedRecoveryTraining.com, along with a list of words that might fit for each of your compass points. Feel free to use words that aren't on the list. The list just gives you a place to start. As you work to create your own compass, consider the work you've done thus far. What do you need to protect yourself from? What tools do you have that you want to rely on as you move forward? As we go through each step, I'll include the words that are currently part of my compass as an example, but please make this your own. There's no wrong way to do this – it's yours.

Draw a circle with two lines crossing through it, one stretching from top to bottom and one from side to side. You can make it as plain or as fancy as you want. Let's start with the middle – what centers you? How do you stay grounded? What anchors your soul? This may relate to people, roles, and responsibilities you have in life, for example your kids or parents or friends. It may be your Higher Power. It may be the big picture of what you're working toward. It may be a philosophy of life or way you're trying to live. I've made several versions of my personal compass. On my most recent compass, the center is "balance." It's very difficult for me to move forward without balance, and when I struggle to make progress, often I need to rebalance the areas of my life.

Now let's move to the north position. What are you moving toward? What is your North Star? The North Star has been used by sailors in the northern hemisphere for thousands of years to guide them safely to their destinations. It stays in the same place, allowing sailors to orient their ships. How do you guide yourself? Is it a goal? A mindset? A philosophy? A personality trait that you are working to develop or strengthen? This can be used when you make decisions in your life as you can ask yourself if the decision moves you in that direction. The last time I created a personal compass, my north was "authenticity." which for me involves connection to myself and others along with staying true to what I feel and know and to who I am.

Whatever you put in the south position of your compass is what drives or pushes you in the direction you want to go. You could also picture this point as what provides the support for you to move forward. What makes it safe? How do you have the strength to continue? For me, this is "connection." I am where I am in my life because of the people connected to me and the support and love they provide.

The east and west points of your compass are what redirect you when you start to get off course. For me, these are "boundaries" and "love," which I find help me to balance my choices. Boundaries without love feels harsh to me, and love without boundaries doesn't feel safe, which highlights that often the east and west points can work together to balance each other out.

Again, there is no wrong way to do this. And you can redo it at a later time if the compass you create now doesn't feel as accurate in the future. If you want to add additional points, feel free to. I chose to add NW, NE, SW, and SE to my compass as there were other words I wanted to include. My additional words are "voice," "truth," "limits," and "wholehearted." When I created the first version of my compass, "wholehearted" was my north. It's shifted for me as I worked to balance my life but is still an important part of my process.

Exercise 2–11:

1. Using the diagram available at ConnectedRecoveryTraining.com, draw your own personal compass.

Super Short Summary:

Therapeutic disclosure of information around betrayal can be helpful but needs to be done in a way that is structured and helpful, rather than shaming. Whether or not you do a therapeutic disclosure, working to understand who you are and who you want to become is an essential part of recovering yourself and directing you as you work through recovery. Exploring who we are includes considering resentments, fears, deception, shame, faulty core beliefs, strengths, abilities, accomplishments, and potential.

Chapter Questions:

1. What did you connect to the most in this chapter?
2. What steps are you taking to apply this material to your life?

3

Boundaries

Accountability

The boundaries component of early recovery means accountability to self and others. We've done the work in Chapters 1 and 2 to see ourselves clearly. We can use that clarity to create boundaries for ourselves and those we are connected to. This is an essential step in creating emotional safety for ourselves and maximizing our connection to self and others. Often the words "boundaries" and "accountability" come across as rigid, harsh, shaming, or punitive. When used in a grounded and healthy way, they aren't any of those. They are freeing and connecting, although they may feel uncomfortable initially.

Merriam-Webster (n.d.-c) defines accountability as "an obligation or willingness to accept responsibility or to account for one's actions." This step in the process empowers us to explore the ways in which we have control of what happens to us and what we want to do about it. It provides us with the ability to continue to make choices for ourselves rather than be pushed into reacting to the choices of others. This is a vital step for each of us.

Exercise 3–1:

1. How would you define the term "boundaries"?
2. What comes up for you as you define it? Do boundaries feel safe? Or punitive? Do they feel accessible? Or completely out of reach? Is there shame connected to setting boundaries for yourself? Is there shame connected to having others set boundaries with you? What emotions would you connect to boundaries?
3. What experiences have you had with them in your life so far? List some boundaries you currently have and if those feel helpful or harmful to you and your relationships.

Boundaries and Trust

Boundaries protect and connect. They are created when we identify our limits, honor those limits, and figure out how to respond when others do not honor them. To explain boundaries to clients when they are in my office, I sometimes have them stand up and try to reach the top of my door frame. Most of my clients can do that, although some need to jump. Then I have them try to reach the iron phoenix above the door. As it's probably eight feet off the ground, very few of my clients can reach it, even if they jump. Then I have

DOI: 10.4324/9781003623359-5

them try to reach my ceiling. It's ten feet tall, so I haven't yet had a client that could reach that. Boundaries are defined when we recognize that we've stretched as far as we can and/or decide how far we are willing to stretch in relationships. You might be able to reach the top of the door frame (metaphorically in a relationship) if you stretch, but having to stand stretched out for years may not be something you're willing or able to do. Defining and implementing boundaries increases connection because it gives us the ability to maintain the level of connection we are offering. If we push to stretch ourselves to the absolute limit of our abilities, we can't hold it indefinitely.

Boundaries with others are related to trust. Trust can be defined as behavior over time, or predictability of outcome. We usually think of trust as being able to rely on someone for something in a positive way. We also usually define trust regarding a person as a whole; when we say we trust someone, we're saying we believe they will be there for us when we need them and will keep our confidences. Trust is often more accurate when the concept is broken down into much smaller pieces. Maybe you can trust that a significant other will be there for you emotionally, but you can also trust that they aren't great at budgeting or keeping up with the laundry. Maybe they are great at communicating with your kids, or advocating for you in situations with your family, but they struggle to communicate with you around physical connection.

When we better understand ourselves and those we are connected to, we can figure out how to set boundaries that maximize our connection with them. For example, when I was a stay-at-home mom, I had a friend who I loved hanging out with. My kids loved hanging out with her too. I found out that she'd shared something I told her in confidence with another friend. It confused me until I stepped back and considered the situation in a different way. I realized she defined protecting confidences differently than I did. She assumed that confidences were kept within our friend circle rather than between the two of us. Once I realized that, I could choose how to address it. I could change my definition of what keeping confidences meant in that relationship, I could talk to her and ask that she shift her definition of keeping something confidential to defining it as between the two of us, or I could stop sharing things with her. If I didn't talk with her about changing the definition, I knew I could trust that information I told her would be shared with our friend group. I could also trust that she loved me and my kids. I could trust that she'd be there in a second if I needed her. I could trust she'd take care of my kids like they were her own. When you can see who people are and create this type of trust, you maximize your ability to connect to them because you make connection safe by knowing how they will respond in various situations. No one is perfect. Boundaries allow human connection.

That doesn't mean you just have to be ok with the ways that are currently safe for you to trust someone. I could have chosen to have a conversation with my friend about the differences in how we defined confidences so that I could have shared information privately with her. In that case, I decided I didn't need to, because I was ok with shifting my definition of keeping confidences to hers in that case. Meaningful and deep relationships often require us to work on changing or communicating changes we need to others to develop trust that feels safer for us and others.

The example I just gave was a less painful one than many of the situations that come up when there has been betrayal, but the boundaries work the same way no matter how painful the situation is. When we are hurt, it indicates that boundaries have been crossed or that we need different boundaries. Examining the situation helps prevent us from being hurt in the same way again. We start by figuring out what boundary was crossed or where we need to put up a new boundary. Then we figure out if we want to change our boundaries to match what was done, if we want to have a conversation with the other person or people to explain our boundaries, or if we need to take steps to protect ourselves. When you set up the boundaries to keep yourself safe, you create a situation where you can choose to stay in the relationship while they do the work to change those responses because you have minimized the way this pattern of behavior can impact you.

One issue that comes up around this topic is deception. Often the boundaries we have are based on how someone else represents themselves and their actions. If someone deliberately misrepresents themselves and their actions, it makes it difficult to know how to define boundaries with them. This is the reason deception is one of the most difficult parts of betrayal. If there is deception, we don't have the information needed to know where to set our boundaries or how to create safety within that relationship. When major deception is part of the equation, we need to set up boundaries that protect us even if the other person lies again. Sometimes that means separating or even ending the relationship. If the deception focuses on one or two aspects of the relationship, finances for example, we can set up stricter boundaries in that area and still work to strengthen our connection to them in other areas. It is not safe to assume that the discovery of deception will prevent it from happening again. We can change patterns, but we need to do the work to understand why that pattern developed and work to develop new patterns. If the person you are connected to is unwilling to listen to how their behaviors are impacting you, there is very little chance that those behaviors will change. You then need to consider what boundaries you need to set up so you will not continue to be hurt by them.

Exercise 3–2:

1. Did the information in the section above change your view of boundaries? Why or why not? If it shifted your view of boundaries, how did your view change?
2. Did the information in the section above change your view of trust? Why or why not? If it shifted your view of trust, how did it change your understanding?
3. Did any stories in your own life come up for you as you read? If so, what did you remember? Process through any emotions with your therapist and/or group.

Communicating Boundaries

Boundaries can be most effectively communicated using the following steps:

1. Start with the underlying message – "I'm having this conversation because I love you and want to be connected to you."
2. Using your emotions and needs, explain your limits – "When _____ happened, the message I got, whether or not you meant to send that message, was _____, which made me feel_____. I know I'm going to struggle to be connected until we sort through it."

3. Explore changes/solutions that might resolve the issue – "Would it be possible to _____? Or are there other suggestions you think might be helpful?"
4. (Optional – primarily used if negative response is received) State the steps you will use to honor your limits if the boundary is crossed – "If we can't come up with a solution that feels safe, I'm going to take the following steps for now and would like to discuss this topic in our next therapy session."

The conversation starts by stating the underlying message. Please note – this isn't just the change you want the other person to make. It isn't even what you feel. It's deeper. It's the reason you're having the conversation, which is usually because you want to be connected to the other person and you're currently feeling disconnected. You're having the conversation because your connection with the other person matters. It usually sounds like "I'm having this conversation with you because I love you and I want to be as connected to you." If the relational dynamics have changed for the better due to recovery work, it's ok to include that in this statement. For example, that might sound like "I'm having this conversation with you because I love you and I really love the connection we are building. I've felt so much closer to you in the last several months and I really don't want to lose that, so I want to work through this."

When we work to express ourselves and heal aspects of relationships that are leading to disconnection, we are making a bid for connection. We seldom fight for connection with people who don't matter to us. When we look at the underlying message first and share that part of the conversation with the other person, we ground ourselves, and hopefully the conversation, in the reality of the relationship. It helps to shift both parties into using the conversation to build connection. This doesn't minimize or dismiss our feelings; in fact, it does the opposite. It reminds us how important it is to be connected to the other person and helps us see that it's important that we work to advocate for ourselves and our relationship with them. It also helps to start the conversation in a way that feels more collaborative, meaning it is less likely to produce a defensive response. When we feel loved and wanted, we are less likely to put up shields. The person who brought up the conversation is more likely to be heard, each person is more likely to feel valued, and it is more likely that you will come up with a solution that resolves the situation.

With that context, we move on to the second step of the process. Using our emotions and needs, we share what it is that we're trying to communicate about and communicate our limits. The most basic format for this is I-statements, a format originally developed by Thomas Gordon (1970). I-statements focus on how we were impacted by something rather than arguing details. "When _____ happened, the message I got was _____, which makes me feel_____." It's important to phrase this from our perspective, sharing about our experience rather than trying to argue our point (as in making a courtroom argument like a lawyer). Context and opinion are the least effective ways of presenting an experience, but they are the most commonly used approaches. Conversations that focus on context and opinion usually turn into arguments about details because details make us feel like we have to agree on every detail to agree on how someone feels about the situation. Using generalized context and focusing on our emotions makes it more likely that we can be heard and understood and move toward resolving the issue. Using I-statements can help us feel more grounded and stay congruent with who we are without giving up on advocating for ourselves.

The third step in the process is exploring changes that might resolve the situation. Asking for the other person's input increases the chance that the other person will hear what you're saying and increases the chance that the two of you can come up with a solution that changes the pattern. If you've already tried to talk about this pattern multiple times, I recommend you bring it to therapy and have your therapist help you work through why those patterns continue to happen.

Finally, step four can be used if the other person responds negatively to your request. If this happens, you don't have to escalate to continue to advocate for yourself. You can stay grounded and state your limits and the steps you need to take to honor those limits. In this case it might sound something like "I'm trying really hard to work with you to figure this out, but it feels like this conversation is escalating and we're spinning. I'm going to save this for our next therapy session and discuss it there."

A handout listing each step of this process is available at ConnectedRecoveryTraining. com.

Exercise 3–3:

1. Think of a time that you were hurt by someone who matters to you (you might want to try to stick with a minor event to practice this).
2. Figure out what boundary or boundaries were crossed. Note that feeling hurt indicates that a boundary was crossed somewhere. It may be on your side – you may have expected something different or may have not communicated something. It may be on their side – they may have crossed a line that made a situation painful or unsafe for you.
3. Think about how you would like the situation to change so you won't be hurt again. Are there steps you want to take (such as me deciding to change what I shared with my friend)?
4. Think about if you would like to communicate with the other person and ask to work together toward change (such as I would do if it was my husband who revealed something I'd shared with him in confidence).
5. Figure out what boundaries you need to set up for yourself. These may be permanent (changing what you expect from a relationship) or temporary (changing what you are doing or sharing until a shift is made that makes it safe to return to the prior way of doing things).
6. Using the format above, write down how you would address the situation with the other person involved.

Three Circles

In order to determine what boundaries we need to set up, we first need to identify the behaviors that are disconnecting. In this stage of recovery, we focus on escape patterns (tied to escape cycles) and incongruent behaviors (which we all have), which I call relational relapses. Let's talk a little bit more about relational relapses. Each of us has patterns and reactions we default to that aren't helpful, connective, or congruent with who we are and who we want to be. Usually these are ways we try to control or manipulate situations or individuals so that we don't hurt. These approaches might make us feel less pain in the moment, but long-term, they usually cause us and those connected to us more pain. Identifying and changing those patterns can help to increase connection and peace in our lives and our relationships. It's not about ignoring the needs behind those behaviors – it's about finding more effective and helpful ways to address them. One way to start that process is to create a "three circles" diagram for them.

Years ago, an SAA group created the concept of the three circles to define healthy versus unhealthy behaviors for each of them. The three circles focus on three different types of behaviors: escape patterns, things that lead to or make us more vulnerable to escape patterns (we call these "indicators" and "triggers" in the recovery process, so you recognize those words when we bring them up in just a minute), and healthy behaviors. This can be generalized and applied to everyone, not just those with significant escape patterns, if we shift it to include relational relapses. If you need a visual format, ConnectedRecoveryTraining.com has worksheets for your three circles for both escape patterns and relational relapses (to honor the work the SAA group that originally came up with these did, along with the work 12 step ministries have done in general, these diagrams have no copyright or logos). If you have patterns of escape behaviors, create a three circles list for both escape patterns and relational relapses.

For escape patterns, the middle circle includes numbing or escaping behaviors. These are behaviors you know are unhealthy and disconnecting for you and are part of your escape patterns. For relational relapses, the middle circle is a list of your relational relapses, or the ways you respond to things reactively and non-congruently.

For escape patterns, the second circle includes warning signs, which includes both triggers and indicators. I'll explain triggers and indicators in just a minute. For relational relapses, this circle includes emotional bucket drainers and triggers. Basically, this circle includes items that push us toward the center circle reactions/behaviors or make it more difficult for us to stay grounded in who we are and who we want to be.

The outside circle includes healthy behaviors we work to add to our lives, both recovery behaviors and emotional bucket-fillers.

Indicators and Triggers

Both indicators and triggers play a part in acting out and relational relapses (see the Recovery Slope Diagram in Figure 3.1). I use the metaphor of building a fire to explain the difference between indicators and triggers. Indicators are wadded up pieces of paper, kindling, or logs. Triggers are lit matches. If you drop a lit match on an empty cement floor, it goes out. If you drop a lit match on a pile of paper and wood, you start a fire. The size of the fire depends on how much paper and wood is on the floor.

Indicators (for both escape behaviors and relational relapses) can be things that happen and have nothing to do with choices we make. It could be not getting enough sleep, or being sick, or stress at work. It could be having several rainy days in a row (if rain depresses you – I personally love rain and it cheers me up, but I think I'm in the minority in that area). It could be that it's the first week or two of school for your kids and they are cranky. In those cases, there's usually not much we can do to change the situation. We work to be

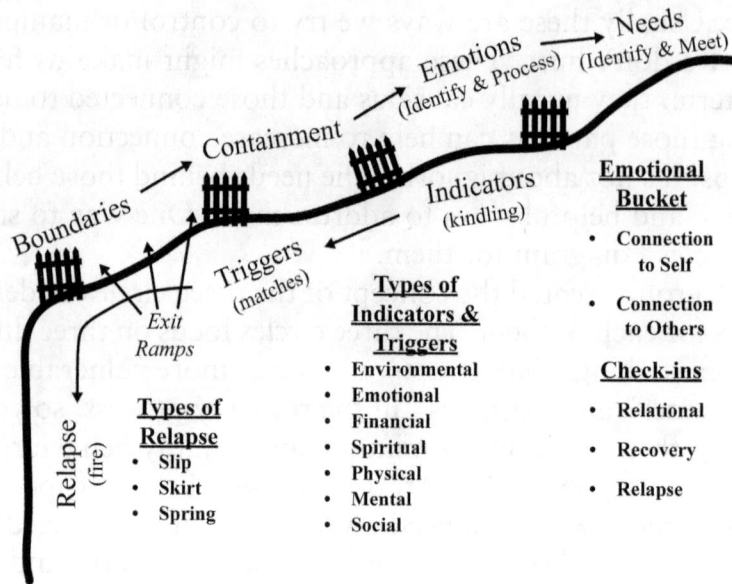

Figure 3.1 Recovery Slope Diagram

aware of the potential impact the situation will have on us, so we have the ability to buffer that effect. For example, if we know a certain time of year is usually super stressful at work, perhaps we can work to minimize other responsibilities during that time. Or maybe plan a vacation immediately before or after to recharge.

Indicators can also be things we do or expose ourselves to that lead to escape behaviors or increase our chances of reacting into a relational relapse. For example, with escape behaviors, we could avoid checking in with ourselves daily, isolate instead of reaching out, or skip individual or group therapy sessions. In the case of relational relapses, it could be not doing the work to set boundaries or deciding to ignore signs that make us feel unsafe.

Triggers (lit matches) are things that send us into relational relapses or activate our desire to numb or escape. They can be things we can predict, like driving by a hotel that was used as part of an affair. They can be things we may not be able to predict, like a smell or word that suddenly brings up a memory connected to either past escape patterns or betrayal or trauma.

Both triggers and indicators can fall into pretty much every category you can think of – environmental, emotional, financial, spiritual, physical, mental, or social. The more information you have about your triggers and indicators, the greater your ability to minimize them or create safety around them.

Exercise 3–4:

1. Create a three circles diagram or list for either escape behaviors or relational relapses or both.
2. What came up for you as you created your three circles? Share them with your therapist and/or group. If you feel comfortable doing so, ask for feedback.
3. Is there anyone it might be helpful to share your three circles with? If you're in a primary relationship, do you feel safe sharing them within the relationship? If you decide to share them, I recommend using a therapy session to do so. If it doesn't

feel safe to do so, talk with your therapist about why that might be and see if there are steps that might make it safe to share. Note that sometimes sharing information such as this can be used as a weapon against us. If you are worried that might be the case, talk through the situation with your individual therapist as that indicates opportunities where additional boundaries might be needed. Also, if you have not gone through disclosure yet, sharing your three circles within your relationship might be triggering if it includes information you haven't shared yet. Work with your therapist to determine how to share your three circles in a way that helps to create safety and build a foundation for connection.

Boundaries List

Exploring our three circles helps us identify the boundaries we have and the boundaries we need to create. Often there are several areas in which boundaries need to be set up. It may be helpful to refer to your three circle worksheets, and possibly the work you and those connected to you did through the disclosure process (review those in therapy if they are willing to share them – do not ask them to share them outside of a therapy session). As with the other tools we've created, it is likely that as you move through the recovery process, this chart will change. You may figure out new disconnecting behaviors, your responses to those behaviors might change, or the reparative action might change.

Exercise 3–5:

1. Create a list of boundaries for yourself.
2. Create a boundaries list for your primary relationship or one of the important relationships in your life.

This tool can be used for relational patterns/relapses, escape behaviors, or any disconnecting behaviors. All human beings need boundaries. No relationship is perfect. As you move through recovery, it is likely that the focus will shift to more relationally disconnecting behaviors rather than escape patterns or trauma responses.

Slips, Relapses, and Making Amends

Despite our best efforts, there will be times we slip into old patterns or are triggered into a relational relapse or pattern or an escape behavior. Planning for perfection is a nice thought but is not realistic and does not create safety for us or those connected to us. I often hear phrases like "I feel so much better now – why in the world would I ever do that again?" or "I'm never going back!" While those may feel true, believing that we can move forward without any hiccups is not helpful. That being said, this isn't meant to be used as an excuse for relapses into painful, disconnecting, and incongruent behaviors. Part of recovery is working to minimize slips and relapses into those behaviors and working to repair them when they do happen.

As we move through recovery, we create boundaries around ourselves and our relationships that allow us to build the life and the connections we want. Those boundaries keep us safe and add joy, peace, and excitement to our lives. It may not make sense that boundaries would do that, but that is what boundaries are for, to create safety and connection. They don't limit us, but rather maximize our access to the life we want. Let's think of boundaries as a fence around our yard. We can make that yard as small or as big as we'd like, provided we can take care of it so it's not dangerous for us. I live in Texas, so if you don't keep your yard mowed, you'll end up with snakes and tarantulas (ick!) in the grass. If you don't keep up on pest control, you'll end up with fire ants. If you want to be able to spend time outside, or let your kids or pets enjoy the yard, snakes, tarantulas, and fire ants prevent that from being safe.

Another issue we may have with keeping our yard safe is gaps in the fence. We got my daughter a puppy for her seventh birthday. We had a six-foot privacy fence around our backyard, so we assumed it would be ok to let him out to run. We didn't realize there was a gap under the gate, which he wiggled through. Fortunately, he just wanted to get back inside with us, so we found him scratching at the front door. We also had problems letting him play in the backyard when the neighbor's dog decided he wanted to play with the puppy and figured out how to knock down pieces of the fence so they could get into each other's yards. We had to put up a stronger fence on that side of the yard so we could make sure it was safe for the puppy and our kids.

We can expand our boundaries as we figure out how to keep that part of our world safe and increase our capacity to care for additional square footage. We also need to figure out where the gaps in our fences are and make sure those gaps are filled. Not because we're trying to limit ourselves, but rather because we're trying to create an environment that is safe for us and those connected to us that we can enjoy without fear.

If you slip back into a pattern you're trying to avoid, or do something that hurts yourself or others, take the time to process through what you did and repair it. Start by reaching out for support. Falling back into old patterns or turning to new reactions that are incongruent indicates that we've hit our limit somehow. This means we need help. We can't do it alone in that moment. Sometimes this means reaching out to a friend or group member. Sometimes it means setting up a therapy appointment. Sometimes it means sitting down and taking steps to reconnect to ourselves, often starting with venting or soothing. One rule of thumb – **do not** look for support from someone you hurt with your behavior. Asking someone you just hurt to support you in the moment, especially before you've done the work to create safety, is not appropriate or connective and will deepen the pain caused. Also, don't go to someone you're mad at to vent or soothe. You will likely just get more upset if you try and talk to the person your anger is pointed at.

It's easier to explain this concept if we switch from emotional pain to physical pain. I'll use a story about my son. We don't get snowstorms very often in Texas, but we get them occasionally. One time when we got a "big" snowstorm (for Dallas), my kids and I went outside and had a snowball fight. I hit my son with a snowball, so he ran up and rubbed snow in my face, then ran away laughing (we were all laughing at that point). He wasn't watching where he was going as I was chasing him to throw another snowball at him, and he slipped and fell and broke his wrist. In that moment, I immediately felt badly that I'd been chasing him. It wouldn't have been helpful or appropriate for me to look to him for support around my guilt. Instead, I needed to help him up and get him first aid for his broken wrist. He was hurting. And it wasn't his job to support me.

In that particular situation, I don't think either of us was at fault. We were both participating in the snowball fight and the slip was a mistake. Sometimes pain (usually trauma triggers in cases like this) will be mistakes like that, where no one involved did anything wrong in the moment or in the past. It's more likely that trauma triggers are directly related to something that was painful in the past (either recent and done by the person involved, or farther in the past and done by someone else). If the pain was caused by us, we often feel shame, guilt, or pain when we see the pain the other person is in. In those moments, we need to recognize that the other person's pain needs to be addressed first, and then we can address our own pain with someone not directly hurt by the situation. Please note, if someone's reaction is abusive, there are ways to acknowledge the pain we've caused without dismissing the abuse.

Outside support (meaning support from people not directly connected to the current situation) can be invaluable in allowing us the space and lack of reactivity to process our emotions and reactions before addressing them with the person, or people, connected to them. It's not meant to decrease the other person's responsibility if they did something that hurt us. It's meant to give us the chance to process through our emotions and present them in a deeper and more complete and congruent manner.

Once we've figured out what support we need and have reached out to people who can help us as we process through what happened, the next step is sorting through how we got to where we got to. Like the previous steps, this step needs to be done without involving the person you were triggered by or the person who you hurt with your escape response. When we process something, we need to give ourselves the space to say things imperfectly and often early steps of processing include blaming someone else. Sorting through that response is necessary before asking someone for a repair. Additionally, healing and empowerment comes from realizing the ways we can change the situation ourselves instead of just relying on others to create safety for us. This isn't meant as a pass for damaging and disconnecting behavior. Those behaviors still need to be challenged and addressed for relationships to grow or become safe.

As we consider what led up to the relational relapse or escape behavior, look for the things you have control over. Look for your part as well as contributing factors from others. This helps us to empower ourselves and creates safety and peace more quickly and at a more complete level.

The next step is to identify the "gaps in our fence" and figuring out how to fill them in. As we discussed earlier, boundaries are fences we build around ourselves so we can safely enjoy the connection and interactions in our lives. Relational relapses or escape behaviors indicate that something got through that fence. Sometimes we need different boundaries around situations or actions. Sometimes we need to process trauma connected to something. Sometimes we need different boundaries around someone else. Sometimes it's a leftover reaction from something that has hurt us before.

As you process through what happened, consider who was hurt by your escape behavior or relational relapse. This includes yourself. If someone was hurt by what you did, then it's important to take steps to repair that pain.

Exercise 3–6:

1. Think of a recent situation in which you slipped into an escape behavior or relational relapse. What type of support did you need?
2. What was going on in your life right before that happened? How did it contribute to the situation?
3. Where was the "gap in your fence"? What steps might be helpful to stop this situation from happening again?
4. Who was hurt by what happened? What steps do you need to take to repair any harm done?

Priorities and Accountability

Looking at pain in your life often includes acknowledging that people you love, admire, and look up to, hurt you or were part of things that hurt you. The point of this work isn't to demonize them. When we start this work, many of my clients worry that I'm trying to tell them their parents were bad parents. While there are cases where parents are abusive and negligent, and in those cases the depth of the responsibility of the parents needs to be considered in the creation of boundaries moving forward, many cases do not involve significant abuse or neglect, just humanness. We still need to process the experiences those clients went through. Just because someone didn't mean to hurt you, or someone did their best, or someone didn't know it was painful for you, that doesn't mean you didn't hurt.

I use this metaphor to explain why we need to look at our pain and how that connects to the role others have played in it. If you and I are in a room and I have a brick in my hand, and at some point the brick leaves my hand and ends up hitting your head and splitting it open, what is the first thing you need to do? Stop the bleeding and take care of the wound. It doesn't matter how the brick got from me to you, you still have a head wound that needs to be taken care of. Once we've taken care of it, the second step is to figure out how the brick got from me to you. Maybe I set it down on a table you happened to be sitting next to, and then I bumped the table and it fell off. In that case, neither of us was at fault, but we probably shouldn't put bricks on tables that people are sitting next to. Maybe I tripped and it flew out of my hand and hit you. In that case, I might need to be more careful, or it may have just been a fluke and there isn't much we'd need to change. In those cases, the boundaries focus more on how to prevent accidents. If I threw it at your head because I was mad at you, that is a different scenario and will take different levels of accountability and boundaries. If I don't do the work to see that it's absolutely not ok to throw bricks at people, then I would recommend you set a boundary that you won't be in a room with me, or if you have to be, you wear protective gear. So, to summarize, the first step is to look at the wounds we have, and the second step is to consider the role others played in creating those wounds.

Exercise 3–7:

1. How can understanding your family of origin's role in your past pain help you create more compassion for yourself in your healing process?

Super Short Summary:

Boundaries protect and connect us. Understanding our limits helps us to know what boundaries we need. Trust is behavior over time. Communication works best if we start with explaining that we're having the conversation because the other person or people matter to us. If you slip back into a behavior you're trying to avoid, explore how you got there and take the steps to repair your connection to yourself and others.

Chapter Questions:

1. What did you connect to the most in this chapter?
2. What steps are you taking to apply this material to your life?

4

Communication
Containment

The next component of the Connected Recovery® process is communication. Communication is often a struggle at this point of recovery. Triggers may be frequent, and connection may be limited. Because of this, communication in early recovery focuses on developing skills around containment, processing, and the format of reconnecting after processing. The primary tool we use for those skills is calling a time-out.

I think most of us are familiar with the concept of time-outs. It's a fairly common practice to have kids take time-outs if they get angry or are mean to someone else. Time-outs aren't just useful for kids though; time-outs are useful throughout life. Not as a punishment, but to give us time to be able to process through something before responding to it. A commonly believed fallacy is that we need to respond to conversations, requests, etc., in the moment. It works to respond to things in the moment if we know how we feel about them and are ok with offering whatever it is that we're offering. Otherwise, it's important to give ourselves time to sort through the situation before responding. The time-out diagram (see Figure 4.1) can help you sort through whether or not you need a break to process.

Time-Outs

A classic anger management technique is considering the intensity of our emotions/responses using the metaphor of a thermometer. I use this for more than just anger – it can help us consider where we are emotionally and determine the needs behind the emotions that cause us to be reactive, either internally or externally.

Realize that any emotion can be overwhelming, not just anger. The thermometer looks at the intensity of emotions and whether or not we're able to stay present with that intensity. Even emotions that are "good" emotions can be overpowering or triggering. For example, if connection has not been safe for you, feeling connection, or feeling seen, may push you to the top of the thermometer. If feeling happy has never been something you could trust, feeling happy may do the same. Don't judge yourself for your reactions to your emotions. If you are overwhelmed by them, take the time to process through why you are overwhelmed and figure out what steps you need to take to make the situation safe for you to connect. The time-out process helps us do that. See Figure 4.1.

DOI: 10.4324/9781003623359-6

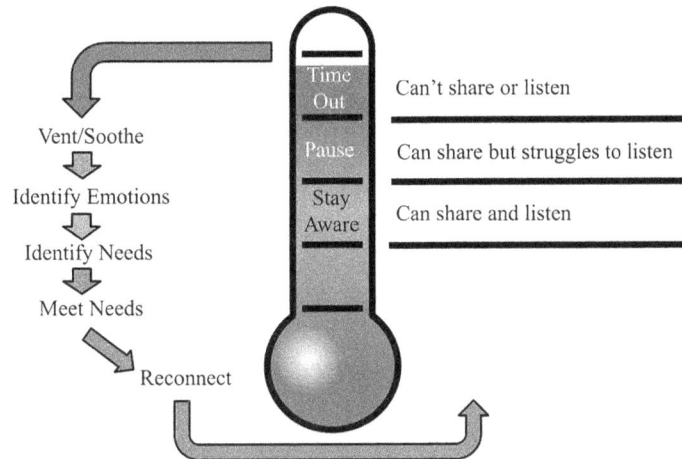

Figure 4.1 Time-Out Diagram

Looking at the diagram, let's start at the bottom of the thermometer. The very bottom of the thermometer (in the full color version of the diagram, this part is green) represents times when nothing is challenging you, nothing is stretching you, and you feel no discomfort at all. We don't live there (at least I don't know anyone who regularly lives there). We may have moments or days or hours where we're there, but most of the time we're in the section above the bulb of the thermometer (this part is yellow).

Exercise 4–1:

1. Can you think of a time when you experienced "green" in your life? When was it?
2. Why do you define that experience as being in "green"? What were you feeling?

The yellow section of the thermometer, which is the section just above the bulb, represents times when we're stretching ourselves and are feeling emotions that are not necessarily completely comfortable but aren't so overwhelming that we struggle to connect or focus. Note that if there's been betrayal, abandonment, abuse, or significant disappointment in your life, even "happy" emotions can be challenging. It can be hard to trust feeling loved or feeling peace if those have not been safe (i.e., if they were used against you or if you experienced a betrayal that made you question reality) or if you haven't regularly felt them. Sometimes those emotions can even be triggering enough that they push us into the orange or red sections of the thermometer. We'll talk about those in just a minute. In the yellow section of the thermometer, you can hear what someone else is saying and you can share what you're feeling. Conversations are reciprocal when each person is in yellow, meaning each of you can be part of the conversation. We need to be aware of what we're feeling and how that's influencing us, so we know if we shift into orange.

Exercise 4–2:

1. What does it feel like for you to be in the "yellow" section of the thermometer?
2. How do you know that you are in a place where you can hear what someone else is sharing?

In the next section of the thermometer (which is orange), we can share what we're feeling, but struggle to listen to someone else share. This often happens when we're afraid we won't be heard or we feel unsafe, but we haven't shifted into a survival response yet. If both people in the conversation are in orange, it's not going to be very productive. At least one person needs to be in yellow for a conversation to be productive. If you're both in orange, then you both need to pause the conversation and do some work to process what you're feeling.

In some cases, we may think the other person is in orange, but they think they are in yellow. Situations like that can be difficult to navigate because telling someone they're in a different color than they think they are is stepping in their hula hoop. We'll talk about hula hoops in more detail in Chapter 8. If your perception is that someone is struggling to hear you, but they say they're in yellow, you can call a time-out for yourself and see if that helps you feel safer. If it happens regularly, I recommend talking with your therapist about how to address it or working on it in a relational therapy session. You can use relational counseling for relationships other than primary relationships. I've had sets of best friends come into my office to work through emotions and patterns in their connection to each other.

In cases where there is betrayal, those healing from betrayal may be pushed into living in orange temporarily because they don't feel safe. If the person who betrayed them can work on learning to stay in yellow, or quickly shift back into yellow, in order to be able to hear their pain and create safety, that can help rebuild trust. This doesn't mean you should force yourself to stay in conversations where the other person is in red, or that you should ignore your emotions and needs. It means if you are able to hear the pain someone is feeling as a result of something you did, you have a higher chance of repairing it more quickly.

If you feel like you're living in orange, realize that staying there drains you very quickly. Relying on someone else to bring you out of orange is not a safe way to live. If you're stuck in orange, work with your therapist to figure out what boundaries you need in order to safely move to yellow. If you're in orange because of something that has been done to you, it will be easier to shift to yellow (and sometimes green) if the person who hurt you works to make amends and heal the situation, but you can do the work to move down the thermometer no matter what the person who hurt you chooses to do.

Exercise 4–3:

1. What signs do you notice in yourself that indicate that you've moved into "orange"? What do you feel? What do you think?
2. What steps can you take to identify when you've moved into "orange"?
3. What might indicate that someone you're talking to is in "orange"?
4. What steps can you take if you believe you or the other person is in "orange" (remember – you cannot call a time-out by telling the other person they are in orange and need a time-out)?

This brings us to the red section of the thermometer. When we hit the red section, survival responses kick in (fight, flight, freeze, frenzy, fold, fawn – see Chapter 1) and we switch into a different section of our brain, the limbic system. If we or the person we're talking to, or both, hit that point, we need to take a break from the conversation because the information isn't being shared in a way that's productive or safe for us or the other person. Sometimes we can hit that point slowly – like the straw that breaks the camel's back. Sometimes we hit that point almost instantly – more like a bubble on the side of a glass of soda (yes, I call it soda, also referred to as pop or coke) breaking free and quickly rising to the top of the liquid and popping. When we are in red, we are unable to think clearly, even if we believe we can or look and sound calm on the outside.

Exercise 4–4:

1. How do you know when you've hit the "red" section on the thermometer? What do you say? What happens internally? What happens externally?
2. How might you be able to tell if the person you're talking to shifts into "red"?

We've talked about how to identify when you might need to call a time-out, namely when you and/or the person you're talking to is in orange or red. Now let's talk about how to call a time-out. It's important to recognize that calling a time-out doesn't mean you're not going to continue the discussion. It doesn't mean you have to stuff your feelings down and pretend they aren't there. It doesn't mean you have to soften what you feel. In fact, processing emotions often allows us to deepen them and share our concerns or pain more accurately. Time-outs are not meant to take away your voice; they are meant to strengthen it.

Time-outs also aren't meant to push something under the rug and prevent it from being addressed. They aren't avoidance. The time-out process is set up to give us a break and the time to process through what we're feeling so we can present it more accurately and cause the least amount of collateral damage as we present it. This approach also helps to balance between the benefits of each side of the pursue–withdraw dynamic while minimizing the costs of each side.

Most interactions between two humans include one person who is more of a pursuer and one who is more of a withdrawer. This isn't bad or good, it just is something we need to be aware of. Pursuers push for issues to be resolved in the moment. They don't want to take a break and process it later because they are afraid the issue will be swept under the rug and won't ever be addressed. The cost of this approach is that interacting when you're both in orange or red means your interactions will likely cause additional pain, which I call collateral damage, and which may damage the relationship more than not finishing the conversation would, at least short-term. While not finishing conversations or addressing issues causes significant long-term damage to relationships, it can be helpful to pause and process before continuing the conversation. Withdrawers push to shut down conversations when they escalate or when the withdrawer feels pressure or discomfort. While this gives both parties the chance to soothe or vent and process, without specific structure, it often results in the issue never being addressed at all. Using therapeutic time-outs allows for the chance to pause, soothe or vent, and process, but also ensures that the issue is addressed and resolved.

Note that you can be both a pursuer and a withdrawer. It may depend on the person you're connecting with. It may depend on the day or topic. Perhaps at work you're more of a withdrawer, but in your primary relationship, you're more of a pursuer. Maybe you're more of a pursuer when it comes to specific topics, but you're a withdrawer in general.

Exercise 4–5:

1. Think of a recent interaction with someone that made you shift into a trauma response or trauma cycle. Go back through the situation in your mind and see if you can tell what color you were when the interaction started. Consider when you shifted into orange, and then into red. Did it happen gradually or suddenly? How did you know you shifted from one into another?
2. Consider the pursue–withdraw pattern. Are you more of a pursuer or a withdrawer? Does that change in different parts of your life? Does that change in different relationships in your life?

Processing Emotions During a Time-Out

Referring back to the Time-Out diagram in Figure 4.1 (the picture of the thermometer), let's shift to the arrows on the left side. Those arrows walk us through the steps of processing out of a trigger or survival response. You can also use the My Trauma Cycle or My Escape Cycle worksheets to complete this step. The arrows on the top of those cycles go through a similar process, although they don't include the first step of the thermometer, actually calling a time-out.

When you're using this process in real time, it's important to start by setting up a specific structure around how you're going to check back in with the other person. We'll talk about how to do that when we walk through the Time-Out Protocol Worksheet (Figure 4.5).

The first step once you've called a time-out (we'll walk through the protocol for calling one in just a minute) is to soothe or vent. Soothing involves internal calming. Venting involves letting the emotion out in order to get to a calmer place. Both can be helpful. Sometimes people prefer one or the other, or it depends on what response you've had. If you have a fight response, venting may be needed, whereas a flight response might respond better to soothing. There's no rule of thumb about what you need though. Go with what feels right for you.

Soothing can include mindfulness, meditation of some type, deep breathing, listening to calming music, etc. Talking to people who help us pause our reactions and calm us down is another type of soothing. Venting often involves physical exertion, like running or hitting a punching bag. It could be listening to music that lets your energy out, like heavy metal or hard rock, or even songs with aggressive or passive-aggressive language. It can also include talking to someone else, provided that the person you talk to doesn't make the situation worse. Talking to someone is soothing if you use that conversation to focus on calming down; it is venting if you use the conversation to get your energy out. In both cases, it **cannot** be the person you are triggered by or upset at. If you are upset at someone or triggered by them, talking to them will not help you to soothe and venting to them defeats the purpose of calling a time-out. Both soothing and venting help to calm and recenter you. I recommend you create a list of 3–5 ideas for soothing and 3–5 ideas for venting. Include options that are available to you in different situations, for example, at work or in the car with your kids, where you might not be able to use the same techniques you can use at home.

Exercise 4–6:

1. Do you usually prefer venting or soothing?
2. What are 3–5 ideas you could use to soothe in each major location you might need to use them in (i.e., at home, at work, in the car, etc.)?
3. What are 3–5 ideas you could use to vent in each major location you might need to use them in (i.e., at home, at work, in the car, etc.)?

Once you've taken the time to soothe or vent, the next step is to figure out what the underlying emotion is. Use the Emotions Circles diagram (Figure 4.2) to try to identify what you were feeling. Focus on specific emotions, not core emotions. Core emotions don't give you enough information to understand what the needs underneath the emotions are. Specific emotions help dig into the core of what we're feeling. When considering what emotions you are feeling, focus on your experience, not on defining what someone else did to you. Note that if you try to do this before soothing or venting, the emotion will be too strong to be helpful. It will just make the situation worse. It's like trying to pick up a hot coal before it cools off.

The underlying emotion can help you figure out what the need is. As we talked about earlier, emotions aren't bad or good, they just give us information about our needs.

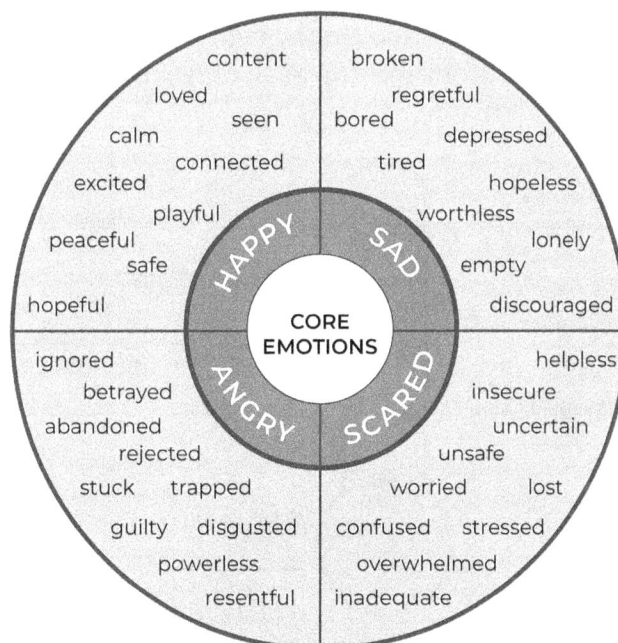

Figure 4.2 Emotions Chart

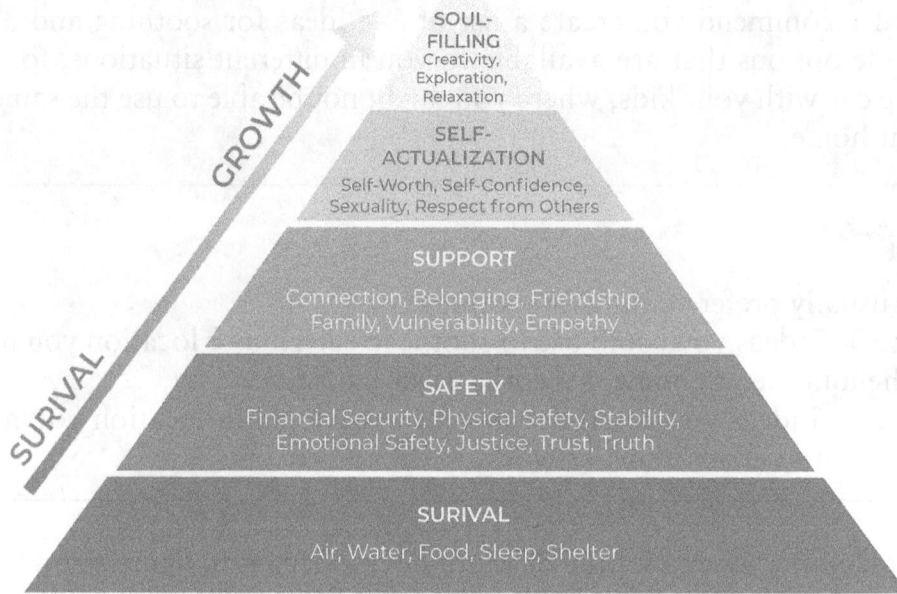

Figure 4.3 Hierarchy of Needs Chart

Needs aren't the solution; the solution is how to meet your need. Needs are more basic than what to do. Use the Hierarchy of Needs diagram in Figure 4.3 to help you identify the need underlying your emotion.

The final step in processing is figuring out how to meet your needs. Start with steps you can take on your own. Identifying the ways you can meet your own needs is empowering and helps to ground you. It decreases desperation related to fear that our needs won't be met by others. This step is not meant to ignore or eliminate what we need from others. It helps to ensure our needs are met on a deeper and more complete level.

I've created a time-out worksheet based on the time-out diagram (see Figure 4.4). You've already completed the work to fill in the top three lines on the right side of the diagram. Use Exercise 4–7 to fill in the left side of the worksheet.

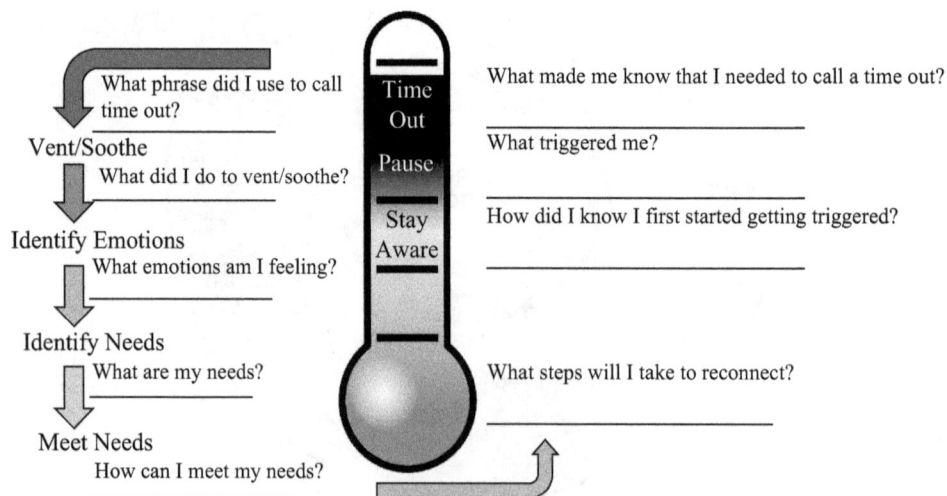

Figure 4.4 My Time-Out Worksheet

Exercise 4–7:

1. Think back to the situation from the previous exercise. When you hit red in that situation, would it have helped to vent or soothe? What steps might you have taken to do so?
2. Using the same situation, use the Emotions Circles (Figure 4.2) to figure out what emotions you were feeling at the time.
3. Use the Hierarchy of Needs (Figure 4.3) to figure out what need was under the emotions you felt.
4. Think about what steps you could take (or took) to meet those needs on your own in a healthy way.

To complete the very last section of the worksheet, you'll need to figure out how to reconnect. Once you've figured out what you can do on your own, decide what you'd like to ask the other person for, or develop a solution together. In most cases, I'd try developing a solution with them over asking them for something specific. Asking for something specific can come across as telling someone else what to do, whereas building a solution with them allows them to be part of the process and allows their needs and limits to be factored in. This is part of the "reconnecting" step.

Exercise 4–8:

1. Using the same situation you've used for the last two exercises, think about how you might talk to the other person about the situation. How much of your processing would you like to share with them? How could you ask for the two of you to work together to come up with a way to resolve the situation?

You can use time-outs in relationships where both of you have worked to set up a structure that builds connection (we'll discuss how to do that in just a minute when we cover the time-out protocol), in relational interactions even when the other person isn't familiar with this tool, or even on your own. To use them with someone who isn't familiar with the process, you can say something like "I'm going to take a break from this conversation, and I'll check back in with you in 30 minutes so we can continue to discuss it." You can change the amount of time you need but always set up a specific time to check back in and then make sure you do so. That doesn't mean you have to be ready to talk or listen in 30 minutes (or whatever time you set up), but if you aren't, then say something like "I'm checking in, but I don't think I've finished processing yet. I'll check back in with you in an hour." Or tomorrow. Or whenever you think would give you enough time. Just make sure that you set up a specific time and you follow up at that time. That helps build trust and makes sure the process gets resolved. If you have to push it out longer than two check-ins, I'd recommend processing it with your therapist or group.

This tool can also be used for individual processing. Recognize that you're in orange or red and take a break from processing. Go through the steps on your own and give yourself time and space to process.

While this may sound like a very detailed process, once you become familiar with the steps, you can use time-outs to process even minor emotional hiccups. For example, if something doesn't feel right to you in a conversation (provided you don't shift into orange or red and stay there), you can quickly pause the conversation and jump through the steps of the time-out process in your head. This helps you to quickly process through what you're feeling and reground yourself. That might sound something like "One second. Let me process this... Ok, I have it more sorted through. Thank you! Keep going." Or it could be even more basic – "One sec... *insert internal processing* ... Ok, thank you! You were saying?" Note that if you can't quickly shift out of orange or red, you'll need to take a longer break to get grounded and figure out what you need, whether or not you choose to share any of your processing with the other person.

Exercise 4–9:

1. What are some steps you could take to pause a conversation for a minute or two with someone you haven't set up a time-out protocol with? What might you say or do?
2. What are some steps you could take to take a break from a conversation with someone you haven't set up a time-out protocol with? What might you say or do?

My Time-Out Protocol

Having reviewed the time-out diagram, let's talk about how to set this structure up within a relationship by using the My Time-Out Protocol Worksheet (Figure 4.5). It's important to have this conversation when each of you are in a calm place. Don't try to set it up in the middle of needing to call a time-out. It may be helpful to set these steps up in a relational therapy session.

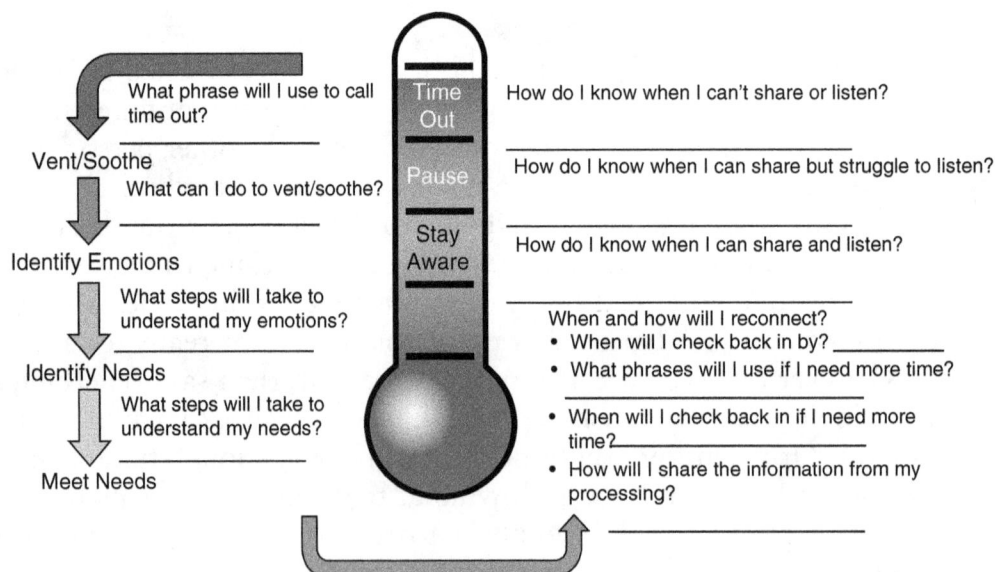

Figure 4.5 My Time-Out Protocol Worksheet

When setting up your time-out protocol, the right side of the worksheet will be filled out by each of you individually. It can be helpful in some cases to share your answers (how you differentiate between when you are in yellow, orange, or red). I'd recommend sharing those in a relational therapy session if possible so you each have support to express any concerns you have.

As we mentioned earlier and will talk about in much more detail in Chapter 9, try to share your concerns without telling them what to do. Also, it can be helpful to start by acknowledging the work they've done and the vulnerability they've shown. For example, something like, "Thank you so much for doing this! I can see you've put a lot of work into identifying when you hit each stage. I know this is vulnerable for me to share, so I imagine it might be vulnerable for you, too. Could I ask if you consider ____ being in orange? My perception is that when you do that, it feels to me like you might be, although I may be off on that."

Also, recognize that you can't just dismiss the concerns you have, even if trying to inter-actively talk about them doesn't resolve them. Pay attention to your gut. If you don't feel like the other person can hear you, check in once or twice, and if the feeling persists, call a time-out for yourself. **Don't** tell someone else you're calling a time-out for them. If this turns into a pattern, discuss it in a therapy session.

Exercise 4–10:

1. Fill in the right side of the Time-Out Protocol Worksheet (Figure 4.5). Consult with your therapist and/or group if needed or if you think it might be helpful.
2. Figure out how much of that side of the worksheet you might want to share within your primary relationship or within the important relationships in your life. Talk with your therapist if you have concerns about sharing parts of it.

The left side of the Time-Out Protocol Worksheet (Figure 4.5) should be shared with any person you're setting the protocol up with. Each of you can decide on how you want to call time-outs. You may just want to use the phrase "time-out." You might want to use a different phrase, like "I need to take a break for a bit" or "I need to pause this conversation for a bit." Do not use "I'm done!" or "This is over" or "Screw you." Those tend to not be quite as connecting, as you can imagine. If you're worried things will escalate (either on your part or someone else's part), then you can use a hand signal. I recommend the classic "time-out" signal with one hand on top of the other, perpendicular to each other, forming a "T." I recommend **not** using hand signals that use a single finger (those may feel validating in the moment but are disconnecting and add more pain to the situation).

The second step on the left side of the worksheet is important for each of you to come up with on your own, and then to share your answers with each other. This helps to address concerns you have and sets up a foundation so it's obvious that each of you are doing what you promised you would do.

In considering what steps you might take to soothe or vent, it can be helpful to discuss who you might vent to. There may be people they would prefer you not vent to. You always have three options when someone asks you to do something; you can say "yes," "no," or "no, but." This applies to someone else telling you they don't want you to vent to someone. They can express their concerns, and you get to decide how you want to respond to that request. You can't choose how they react to your response but you get to make the decision that's right for you. If you tell them you don't care if they're uncomfortable with who you choose to vent to, they may not feel as safe with you. You get to decide the steps that are right for you and they get to decide the steps that are right for them.

It can also be helpful to discuss the physical steps you might take when venting or soothing. For example, if you need to leave the house when you call a time-out, you may need to coordinate around childcare. Or you may want to let them know where you're going so your leaving doesn't cause more trauma.

The next two steps may be similar for each of you. Whether you choose very different processes or similar ones, sharing the steps you're committing to taking and then taking those steps helps to rebuild trust. How are you going to process through your emotions? Maybe use the emotions chart? Or is there something else you connect better to? How are you going to identify your needs? The Hierarchy of Needs (Figure 4.3) chart is my default, but you may have a different process that works for you.

Finally, you need to decide what steps you're going to take to reconnect after you've processed. As we talked about earlier, it's important to have a specific time and way you're going to connect when you call the time-out. This helps to ensure that the issue actually gets addressed instead of avoided. I recommend defaulting to checking in via text after 30 minutes, but you can figure out what format and timing work best for you.

Checking in doesn't automatically mean you're done processing and ready to talk. It can mean that if you're ready to talk. It can also mean you've realized it's going to take longer than 30 minutes to process through the issue. In that case, set up a specific new time to check in. If you think you might be ready in another hour, you might say "I still need more time. Could we check back in an hour, at ____?" As you process, you might realize that the issue is more painful for you than you initially thought, and you really want to check in with your therapist or group first. In that case, you might say "I need to check in with my therapist about this. I have an appointment with them on _____. Could we check in that night at ____?"

Each of you needs to feel ready before you return to the conversation. If one person says, "I'm ready to continue our conversation," but someone else says, "I need more time," then the person who needs more time sets the next check-in time. If the process takes more than a day or two (unless you're waiting for a specific instance, like a therapy appointment), you might want to bring this conversation up in your next relational therapy session or even set up a therapy session to address it. Additionally, if you've tried to have the conversation and had to stop it twice, I recommend defaulting to bringing it to therapy.

Exercise 4–11:

1. Review the left side of the Time-Out Protocol Worksheet (Figure 4.5). Complete each section. Work with your therapist or group if you need help sorting through how to take each step.
2. Set up a time (I recommend a relational therapy session) to share your answers on the left side of the worksheet. If you have concerns about doing so, talk with your therapist and/or group to determine how to make the situation feel safer for you.

Fear Cycle Worksheet

There's one more worksheet that may be helpful in processing through escalating emotions. Often high levels of energy connected to emotions are directly related to fear. I find that many of my clients don't like saying they are afraid of something, so they have a hard time recognizing when fear is part of the equation. Fear can be worry or anxiety. It can be hesitancy. It can be concern about moving forward. Of course, it can be being scared, or even terrified, to do or say something. It doesn't make you weak to feel fear. As with all emotions, fear gives us information. It tells us we may be missing something about a situation, or that a situation isn't currently safe for us. Pay attention to your fear, just like every other emotion.

There are some cases where fear can make us spin. Ironically, this often happens when we are afraid of feeling fear. Additionally, it can happen when we don't know what to do with fear when we feel it. Either way, knowing how to ground yourself when you feel fear is important. The Fear Cycle Worksheet (Figure 4.6) helps you walk through those steps.

It starts with having you identify what you're afraid of. Remember, the word "afraid" may not be the word that occurs to you. It might be "worried" or "anxious" or "concerned." Whatever the wording is that fits best for you, this step helps you identify what your emotions are focused on.

Once you've identified the foundational issue, consider what story you're making up in your head to go along with your fear. Fear often leads us to spin, and like a tornado, we pull in ideas that get scarier and scarier the longer we spin. Sometimes the story we make up is based on things that have happened in the past. Sometimes it is based on things we're afraid will happen in the future. Sometimes it focuses on things we're afraid are already happening. When we take the step to write down the story, we can use that information to recenter ourselves.

Recentering involves taking the story we've written down and grounding ourselves in reality. Maybe things that happened in the past won't happen again because we've changed our boundaries or who we're connected to. Maybe they might happen again, but we've learned to protect ourselves from them. If the story is about the future, consider the worst **plausible** scenario. Figure out how you would survive it. Chances are that you already have the tools to do so or you have the ability to develop them. If the story focuses on something we're afraid is already happening, consider how likely it is and how it might affect us. Taking these steps helps us to process through fear and figure out what we need to do to build safety for ourselves.

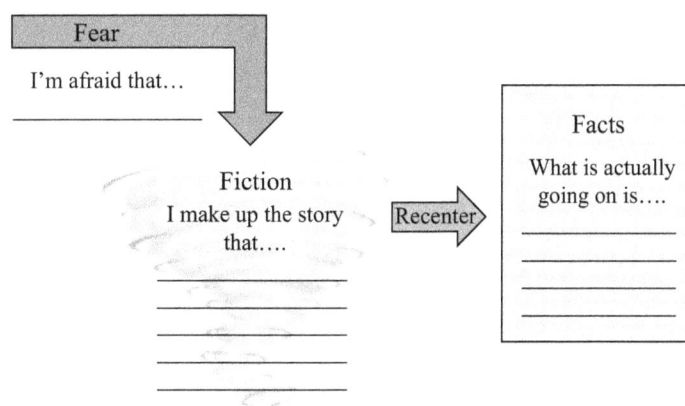

Figure 4.6 Fear Cycle Worksheet

For example, I've had several clients who used these steps to process through fears related to their significant others cheating on them again. In this situation, I'm going to focus on those clients whose significant others proactively leaned into recovery. We'd walk through their fear, which was very valid as they had been betrayed before. They'd realize that they made up the story that they wouldn't be able to tell if their significant others returned to their behaviors. We'd go through the changes they'd seen in their significant others since they started the recovery process. When someone leans into recovery, their whole approach to life changes. Their attitudes, their tone of voice, the way they address things, the concern they show. My clients would detail the differences they saw. We'd talk through the reactions my clients would have when pieces of the person their significant other used to be showed up. They would recognize that they've done the work, and their significant other has done the work, so their interactions are completely different now. My clients would realize that they'd see the changes now if their significant other shifted back into being who they used to be. They also realized that they have steps set up to protect themselves if that were to happen, so they wouldn't be destroyed again.

Exercise 4–12:

1. Think of a situation in which you felt, or feel, scared, worried, afraid, or anxious about something. Use the Fear Cycle Worksheet (Figure 4.6) to walk through that emotion, considering what the stories are that you make up in your head, and what the facts around the situation are. Discuss your experience with your therapist and/ or group.

Super Short Summary:

Sometimes it's helpful to pause, process, and reground ourselves in order to communicate more effectively and authentically. Time-outs can help with that process. Coming up with a specific time-out protocol helps increase our ability to use this tool.

Chapter Questions:

1. What did you connect to the most in this chapter?
2. What steps are you taking to apply this material to your life?

5

Connection

Foundational Connection

The final component of each phase of recovery is communication. In early recovery, communication is often challenging, so we start with check-ins. Check-ins help you share in a structured way. They build a foundation for more vulnerable sharing later in the process. There are three general types of check-ins: relational, recovery, and relapse. We'll go through each type in detail and walk through how to set them up. There are two handouts related to check-ins available at ConnectedRecoveryTraining.com. One describes the three types of check-ins. The other is a worksheet that helps you determine the format that will be used for each check-in. We'll walk you through understanding each type of check-in in this chapter.

Relational Check-Ins

Relational check-ins are the shortest and easiest of the three types of check-ins. They help form a basic connection between two or more people. If you've attended a therapeutic process group with a check-in, they are probably somewhat similar to the process group check-in. It's sharing basic information in a way that gives a general idea of what your day has been like or what you're going through. If you are not currently in a primary relationship, I recommend you set these up with a friend to practice. Learning to share on a regular basis is essential to building connection.

The most basic version of a relational check-in is something along the lines of highs and lows. What was the best part of your day? What did you struggle with the most today? These questions tend to spark more detailed answers than asking "How was your day?"

Communication needs to be balanced for it to be connecting. It can't just be communicating problems or concerns, nor can it be ignoring them and only communicating about "good" things. Communication helps us see others. We are often taught to communicate only about the good or only about the bad. Some of us have been taught to avoid conflict and therefore really struggle to share painful or challenging aspects of their lives or relationships. Others have been raised to believe that "if it ain't broke, don't fix it," which, in regards to communication, really means "if it ain't broke, don't bother bringing it up." We need to hear positive things as much as the painful things. We need to celebrate our wins as well as work on the things that are uncomfortable for us. In order to deepen our connection to others, we need to give positive feedback, so others know if something is being

DOI: 10.4324/9781003623359-7

helpful or connecting, and challenging feedback so that changes can be made to improve connection.

Relational check-ins help start rebalancing connection. Start slow. When you first start using relational check-ins, don't use them to share painful or challenging feedback about the other person. Use relational therapy sessions for that until more healing has happened. Be careful about sharing lows related to something that was said or done. It's important to be able to get to a point where that information is shared, but it's hard to develop this skill if you're also working to keep your shields up. At the beginning of the recovery process, it's often easier to start by sharing highs related to each other. If you find that triggers you or them, process through those emotions in a relational counseling session or possibly in individual counseling sessions.

Set a specific time each day for relational check-ins. Figure out what format works best for you. These can be done in person, over the phone, or even through text. I recommend trying to do them in person, if possible, but if that's challenging or triggering right now, use a different format.

Exercise 5–1:

1. Figure out what format you would like to use for relational check-ins. Are you going to share highs and lows? The best part of your day and the most challenging?
2. When are you going to share these check-ins? Set a specific time each day, and possibly a specific place if needed.

Recovery Check-Ins

Recovery check-ins, like relational check-ins, are also scheduled. They are usually only once a week though and are longer. One of the issues with relational work in recovery is that often it seems like you are supposed to just trust that others are doing their recovery work and moving forward. It can be difficult to trust that that is happening, especially if betrayal is part of your history. Lack of communication can significantly increase triggers for one person or for each of you. Also, this tends to foster walking down your own path without creating a path that you can walk together.

A pattern I often see in recovery is that the person who has been betrayed ends up in a position where they have to push for information, and it feels like they are the parent or a teacher/principal or the detective. As you might imagine, this significantly influences the power dynamics within the relationship and makes it difficult for both to feel connected or safe.

Recovery check-ins help to change the pattern I outlined above. Those who have betrayed are **choosing** and **offering** information, not being forced to share it. They are sharing the information to help rebuild trust and heal the relationship. And those healing from betrayal are also able to share information in a balanced way.

Recovery check-ins help to rebuild trust in the relationship, rebalance the power dynamic, and increase connection. They are longer than relational check-ins. Again, I recommend focusing on doing recovery check-ins once a week. If you find you want to incorporate them more often, you can do so. I don't recommend doing them much less than once a week (maybe every other week, tops), but I also wouldn't recommend doing them each day as that could be exhausting.

Recovery check-ins give you the chance to share the steps you're taking with each other. In a recovery check-in, you share what you did that week. You can share if you had a therapy session or attended group or both. You can share what step of the 12-steps you're working on (if applicable) or what you're currently focusing on. You can share progress and struggles.

The details you share will differ depending on where you are in the process and what you feel is connecting. I have clients who want to talk about every detail of their therapy sessions and clients who don't want to share anything related to therapy. In general, I recommend you start by sharing on a more general level. In early recovery, individual processing is often triggering to talk about. Work with your therapists to determine what feels safe for you. If someone is triggered by the level of sharing (whether it feels like too much or too little), work with your therapists to adjust what you're sharing and how you're sharing it until you find the balance that fits for you and your relationship.

Please remember that if you are attending any type of group (therapist-led, 12 step, or support group), confidentiality is essential to maintain. If you choose to share what you learned from group, you can share the concepts or the emotions you experienced, or what you shared with the group. You cannot share identifying details about anyone in group or details about what other group members shared.

Exercise 5–2:

1. Work with your individual therapist to figure out what you might like to share in your recovery check-ins. Process through any concerns or fears you have about taking this step.
2. In a relational counseling session, work with your significant other to decide what the two of you will share in your recovery check-ins.
3. Set a specific time and day each week (start with once a week unless you have a specific reason to change that timing) for your recovery check-in.

Relapse Check-Ins

Relapse check-ins are not scheduled because they only happen if there is something to share about a relapse into escape patterns or relational relapses. The behaviors shared in relapse check-ins are usually those in the center (red) circle of your three circles worksheets. You can share relapses into either escape cycles or relational relapses (both sets of your three circles). Proactively sharing relational relapses helps to build trust and deescalate relational chaos. It also helps those patterns to change more quickly. Note that for either set of your three circles, you may also decide to share some behaviors from the yellow circles.

Work to develop a format that is not punitive or triggering. Sharing a relapse check-in is not meant as a punishment. It's meant as a step toward ownership and repair. It's something you can offer to help rebuild trust. It often seems counterintuitive, but identifying and sharing when you've slipped back into behaviors you are trying to avoid before you get "caught," or before those behaviors are discovered, helps those healing from betrayal to not have to wonder what is going on that they are unaware of. It's an essential part of building a foundation of trust that helps make hypervigilance unnecessary and connection safe. Following betrayal, those who have been betrayed often worry that something is going on that they don't know about. Sharing relapses, even when they will upset your partner, helps to change the dynamics so that they don't have to wonder if you're hiding something.

Relapse check-ins are vital to relational recovery, and often to individual recovery for both those who have betrayed and those healing from betrayal. Recovery in general is becoming whole again; relational recovery is the relationship becoming whole, connected, and safe. It is not safe to be connected to someone in a relationship where you don't know what's going on. You're always afraid your world is going to be blown up again. You're wary all the time, looking for signs that something is happening. It's exhausting and draining.

Healthy relationships include consent. In this case, I'm not focusing on sexual consent (although that's essential of course – we'll talk about that in much more detail in Chapter 12); I'm focusing on consent in general. Consent requires that all parties are aware of risks, consequences, and benefits (GlittersaurusRex, 2021). Escape patterns and deception take away the ability to choose the relationship, because a clear picture of what the relationship entails isn't offered. Abuse does the same thing. Escape patterns and deception rob each person in a relationship of connection.

Using deception (overt or covert lies), robs yourself of connection and safety. If you are hiding parts of yourself or things you are doing, you'll never know if you are being chosen and loved for who you are. You'll live with some level of constant fear of being found out and rejected. It's incredibly difficult to believe in yourself and your worth in that state. For those being deceived, connection is very challenging. It's difficult to feel safe and relax your guard. In either position, it's hard to feel peace and trust any connection you experience.

For those who have betrayed, it is often difficult to make the leap to proactively share and to believe that sharing will build connection. As we talked about in Chapter 1 when we discussed trauma and escape cycles, healthy behaviors take work in the short term but provide long-term payoffs. Reporting relapses is a perfect example of that concept. Proactively sharing relapses will likely result in short-term pain. It's painful to share, it's painful to hear, and working through the response is painful as well. However, it is necessary to build long-term trust and deep connection.

As we talk about relapse, it's important to identify that there are two types of relapses – escape behaviors and relational relapses. We talked about this earlier when we discussed the two sets of three circles. Escape behaviors include "acting out" into our escape cycles. This can include anything from downloading an app when you committed to avoiding it, to viewing porn (if that's on your list of inner circle behaviors), to contacting a previous affair partner, etc. Anything that's in the inner circle of your three circles for escape behaviors.

Relational relapses are shifting into behaviors that are disconnecting or hurtful. This might mean getting defensive when your partner is triggered. It might be not taking the steps to share who you're going to dinner with, if that's a boundary you've offered to rebuild trust. These behaviors aren't "acting out" or escaping, but they often are disconnecting and can be scary and triggering for your partner.

As we discussed earlier, all human beings have relational relapses. These are attempts to control or manipulate a situation and are behaviors that are incongruent with who you want to be. A benefit of doing recovery work is that you get the chance to identify and change disconnecting patterns. This tool will help you do so. Consider your disconnecting patterns and what steps might be helpful in identifying those and potentially sharing them within your relationship in order to strengthen your connection with yourself and with others and in order to work toward who you want to be.

Often someone closely connected to you will see or react to your relational relapses before you realize you've slipped into one, because they usually involve relational interactions that are triggering or painful for others. Because others may see the relational relapse first, proactively reporting that type of relapse isn't quite the same. Usually with relational relapses, it's more along the lines of owning it and processing the reactions others have to it. The exception to this is deception. Deception might not be seen or sensed in the moment, so working to resolve a situation involving deception would likely involve admitting to it first.

Relapse check-ins are more complex than the other two types of check-ins. Deciding what to share and how to share it can be unsettling, triggering, and scary for each of you. I highly recommend working with your therapists throughout this part of the process and discussing the details of setting up relapse check-ins in cotherapy or in a relational therapy session. We'll talk about how to sort through that in just a minute.

Exercise 5–3:

1. Work with your individual therapist to review your three circles (either escape behaviors and relational relapses, or just relational relapses if you don't have patterns of escape behaviors). Consider what might be helpful to share/report relationally.
2. Process through any concerns or fears you have about taking this step.

Responding to Triggers

Before we go into the steps to set up relapse check-ins, let's talk about how to respond when someone is triggered. These steps are specifically for situations where triggers have been created by betrayal, or when the trigger is sparked by a relational relapse. However, these steps also work to respond to anyone who is triggered. This process is basically the amends process, which may have been used in your therapeutic disclosure process, and which we talked about in Chapter 3. A diagram outlining the steps below is available at ConnectedRecoveryTraining.com.

The first step is to **validate** the fear in the person's response. They aren't crazy. They are triggered because something is showing up and telling them the situation isn't safe.

I recommend overtly saying something like "You aren't crazy. Being upset totally makes sense." Because it **does** make sense. Our emotions are valid. We feel them for a reason. This is a good response to anyone triggered by any situation, whether we're connected to it or not, although it can be a difficult step to take. It often means we need to figure out how to react in a completely different way than we normally do. Don't minimize. Don't be defensive or try to logically argue someone out of feeling their emotions. Don't try to "fix" the situation, because we want them to stop hurting. Telling someone they shouldn't feel that way doesn't help. You can't stop someone from feeling a painful emotion. Don't make it about you. Don't shut down. Sit with them in the pain if you are able to. Taking this step is the beginning of shifting into empathy. It's trying to see a situation through their eyes.

The second step is to **own** your part in creating the wound that was triggered, if your actions either contributed to the current situation, or if your previous actions helped to create the initial wound that this response is in reaction to. This might sound like "I'm so sorry my actions have created this wound in you" or "I'm so sorry that I scared you." Taking this step helps you understand the depth of the impact escape behaviors and betrayal can have on someone connected to you. If the trigger isn't related to anything you did this time or in the past, **empathize** with the person. This sounds something like "I hate that you're hurting" or "This situation must be really unsettling/scary/triggering for you."

The third step is to **offer** to help in a way that might decrease the pain. If the trigger is related to something you did, that might sound like, "Can I share ___ with you? Would that be helpful? What type of support do you need?"

Please note that these responses are NOT meant to be used in abusive situations. If the response is abusive, the only safe response is to exit the situation.

Exercise 5–4:

1. Think of a recent situation in which you were triggered. Using the Validate/Own/ Offer/Ask format, consider what responses might have felt supportive to you.
2. Think of a recent situation in which your significant other or a close friend was triggered. Using the format we just discussed, consider how you responded to them and what you might have done differently.

Steps for Relapse Check-Ins

First, you need to define what constitutes a relapse for you, into either escape behaviors and/or disconnecting relational patterns. The same format is used for both escape behaviors and relational relapses. The list of the behaviors that you're offering to share is a living document, meaning you can add behaviors to the list once you discover they would be helpful to address using this format. You can refer to the inner circle (red) and even the yellow circle of both your three circles (your relational relapses and your escape cycles) for ideas of what to include initially. This step needs to be considered relationally as well. What information might be helpful for you to share? It may include information that doesn't directly relate to escape patterns but might help build trust.

As we discussed earlier, this is not a punishment. It offers information to create safety in areas that have previously been made unsafe. It shows that they matter enough for you to be honest with them. It shows that you're working to change the previous patterns. It shows that they will be allowed to have emotions around mistakes you make and that you aren't trying to hide anymore.

Remember that you always have three options anytime someone asks you to do something (in this case to share something). You can say "yes," you can say "no," or you can say "I can't do that, but I could do this." Also realize that you don't have control over how your response might make the other person feel. If a significant other asks you to share something with them and you say "no," that might affect your relationship with them. But don't agree to share something you won't share. That's deception and will hurt your relationship.

That doesn't mean that sharing relapses will be fun or immediately connecting. Like many aspects of recovery, and many aspects of healthy connection in general, this is often initially painful (short-term cost, long-term payoff). Those you share with may have a strong reaction. They may be upset or hurt or scared or mad. But both of you are showing up in real time in the relationship.

It's not just important to set up structure around **what** will be shared, it's also important to set up structure around **how** the information will be shared. Once you've determined what to share, the next step is to decide how and when to share the information. It's usually essential to have each of you work together to determine what format would be most helpful. I would start by asking them what format they prefer and what scheduling details would be helpful to factor into the equation. Do they prefer face-to-face? Text? Email? Would they like the information to be shared ASAP? Or later that night after the work day is over? What about if one of you are on a business trip or a vacation? Also consider what details will be shared. Often, it's helpful to include the behaviors and the length of time involved, but there may be other details that are needed for your relationship.

In general, I recommend that all relapses be shared within 24 hours or before sex, whichever happens first. Different relationships will prefer different methods of sharing the information. Timing is important to consider as well. For some, knowing immediately is essential. For others, it's important to wait to share until they have time to process or reach out for support. Work within your relationship and with your therapists to determine what feels right for each of you. In some cases, the 24-hour rule may not be helpful. For example, if one of you is on a business trip it may be best to wait until each of you are home to disclose the information. I had one client who was in the middle of a difficult pregnancy when we set up the boundaries for them. She asked that she not be told about any relapses until two months after delivery. We set up structure around that so they both felt safe with the situation. In that case, her husband told his therapist about relapses. That was the right format for them.

To review, so far, we've determined what information constitutes relapse and warrants a recovery check-in, the format that will be used to share that information, and what scheduling details will be factored into the equation. The next step is to determine what details would be helpful to share as part of the check-in. It's important to include enough detail so that the other person knows what happened, while not including unnecessary specific details. The details included will likely differ depending on the specific behavior and depending on what fits best for you. Work with your therapists to figure out what would be helpful and/or necessary for you to share in order to build and maintain trust in your relationship regarding each behavior on your list. Some of the information may be the same for several behaviors. Others may be completely different.

Once you've determined what to include and how to convey the information, come up with a structured format for how the receiving person will respond. My default is to have those receiving the information ask any **clarifying** questions (**not** processing questions), then say, "thank you for telling me," followed by a 24-hour time-out. This format provides time to process without having to provide emotional support to the person who relapsed or responding reactively to the information that was shared. It also gives the person who relapsed time to process what happened and why it happened. This isn't done to prevent natural consequences related to what happened. It isn't done to soften the emotions of those who received the information. Processed emotions aren't softer, they are more direct and more powerful.

The final step is sorting through what steps the person who relapsed will take to process what happened, what they can do to fix it, and what they can do to prevent it from happening in the future. This also includes what they can do to help create safety throughout the process and how the information will be conveyed once they do the work to determine what happened and why it happened. Having a basic format to use is often very helpful as it means you don't have to think about what to do.

The time-out process (see Chapter 4) can be helpful around coming up with a format to check back in once the person who relapsed has completed the work to process through the situation. Continual check-ins help create trust that the situation isn't being swept under the rug. If it takes you longer than 24 hours to process through the relapse, check back in and let them know you're actively processing. Set a future time to check in with them again. Just like with the time-out, if it takes you longer than two check-ins to process, I'd recommend bringing it to therapy.

Exercise 5–5:

1. Using the Check-In Worksheet (available at ConnectedRecoveryTraining.com), work with your individual therapist to consider some ideas for how to address relapse check-ins.
2. In a relational counseling session, share what you are committing to reporting. Define what relapse includes for you, using both sets of your three circles if you have escape patterns and the relational relapse three circles if you don't. Work together to decide what format might be helpful, what details will be included, and how the response might look.
3. Review the Check-In Worksheet and work with your therapists to make sure that both of you have worked together to fill in each section, using the answers from the exercises in this chapter.

Super Short Summary:

Different types of check-ins can be helpful in creating a foundation for communication and connection. Relational check-ins help you share daily experiences. Recovery check-ins including sharing about your recovery process. Relapse check-ins focus on proactively sharing information about returning to behaviors that are damaging for you or others.

Chapter Questions:

1. What did you connect to the most in this chapter?
2. What steps are you taking to apply this material to your life?

Phase 2

Reconnect – Deepening Empathy and Connection

6

Education

Emotions and Needs

Early recovery focused on creating emotional safety through truth. Keep in mind that emotional safety for yourself is possible whether you created it on your own or those you're connected to do the work and help create emotional safety within your relationship. Once you have a safe foundation, the next part of the process focuses on deepening your connection with yourself and others. We'll go back through the five components of the Connected Recovery® model (Education, Honesty, Boundaries, Communication, and Connection) and apply them to middle recovery tools. The education component of middle recovery focuses on understanding your emotions and needs.

Emotions

Emotions in general often get a bad rap. Many of my clients prefer to talk about what they think rather than what they feel, and roll their eyes when I ask, "what emotion is connected to that?" Emotions can seem like an annoyance, because focusing on them often makes us aware of our pain and doesn't initially seem to help alleviate the pain.

Emotions are actually very helpful. They aren't bad or good – they give us information that helps us figure out what we need to do (Plutchik, 2001). Emotions are similar to physical sensations. If I touch a hot stove, it hurts. My nerves send a signal to my brain telling me that the cells on my fingers are being damaged. In response, my body pulls my hand away from the surface so my body doesn't get more damaged. If the burn is bad enough, I'll develop blisters that cover the damaged cells, helping to protect them as they heal. Touching blisters hurts because the cells aren't healed enough to not be damaged if they are touched.

Emotions send us messages just like physical feelings do. The most complete set of information about a situation will come from a combination of our heart and our head. We can't just focus on what we think; we need to consider what we feel and combine that information with what we think to come up with the best solution.

Often it can seem counterintuitive to consider our feelings because they make the pain more obvious. If we can just think our way through something, or even try to ignore it, maybe we won't have to hurt. Feeling our emotions is the only way to heal the pain, which allows us to be happy and connected and feel peace.

DOI: 10.4324/9781003623359-9

Core Emotions vs. Specific Emotions

Emotions fall into two categories: core and specific. Core emotions are valid, but they won't give you enough information to identify the need behind them. It's similar to telling a doctor "I hurt." The doctor needs much more information to understand what's wrong. They need to know what part of you hurts, what type of pain it is, how severe the pain is, and other information.

Studies agree on four core emotions: happy, sad, scared, and angry (Tracy & Randles, 2011). Every model adds additional core emotions, but they don't agree on which ones to add, so we're sticking with those four. These are general categories that emotions fall into. Specific emotions give us more information. Specific emotions are descriptive, they aren't just synonyms for a general emotion. I most commonly hear clients use synonyms for "anger" when I ask what they're feeling. Clients will say "frustrated," "annoyed," or "irritated" rather than the specific emotion related to anger. Specific emotions convey some of the "why" behind the core emotion. For example, if angry is the core emotion and trapped is the specific emotion, you likely feel anger because you feel trapped in a situation or pattern. The emotions chart in Figure 6.1 details specific emotions divided into the four core emotion categories.

Specific emotions are deeper. They help us to connect to ourselves and others at a deeper level. Connection to ourselves deepens because we better understand what we're going through. Connection to others deepens for the same reason and because deeper emotions help to express how situations are impacting us rather than our translation of what someone else is doing. The more we can focus on how we're being impacted by the situation,

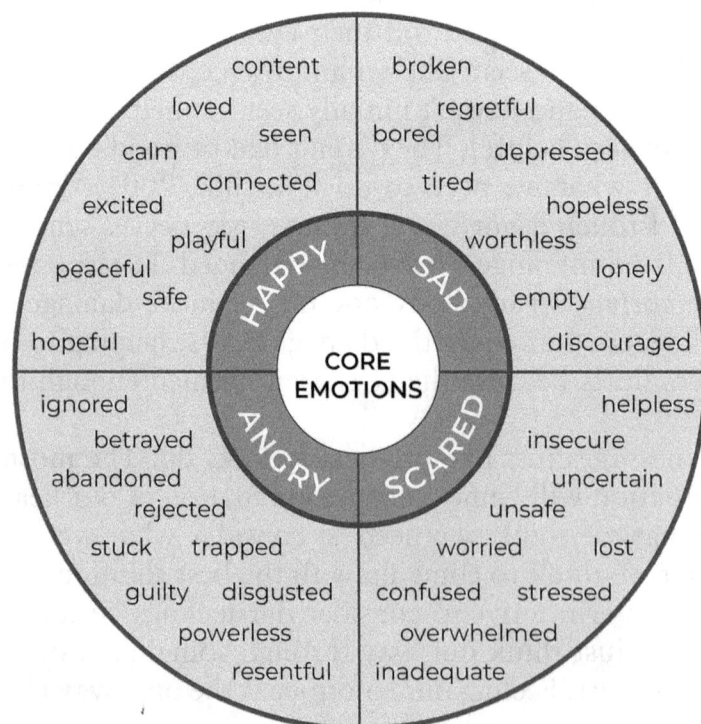

Figure 6.1 Emotions Chart

the easier it is for someone else to hear us. Most people tend to focus on explaining what they believe happened rather than how they feel about it and the messages they got from the situation. If a discussion is about context, meaning what happened, then each person in the conversation needs to agree about exactly what happened, which they won't do. So much time is spent focusing on specific phrasing and the timeline of the situation that there is no bandwidth for understanding what the situation felt like, and the conversation doesn't help resolve the pain.

The next step after identifying the specific emotion is understanding the need behind it. The term "need" is often misunderstood. There is a difference between need and solution to meet the need. The need is more general. See Figure 6.2.

The format Maslow (1943) developed for his Hierarchy of Needs explained that we have to have our more basic needs met to be able to focus on the next level of needs. When considering needs, it's important to recognize two things. One is that "needs" aren't confined to something that keeps us alive. Those are basic needs – the very bottom of the triangle. The other thing to remember is that we need to balance our needs with the needs of those around us. This concept applies in both directions. We can't sacrifice basic needs of our own to try and meet less basic needs for others ("don't light yourself on fire to keep someone else warm"), and don't put your higher level needs above the more basic needs of those connected to you.

As each level of the triangle gets filled in, we move up to the next level. This can show up in our relationships and can indicate progress. When we feel safe with someone, we naturally want to deepen our connection to them.

Considering needs prior to considering solutions allows us to identify more accurate solutions and often broadens the solutions we develop. For example, if I'm struggling, look at the emotions chart and decide that "lonely" is the emotion connected to that pain, the need behind that might be "connection." Solutions that meet that need might include spending time with my husband, hanging out with my kids, or going out with friends. This allows me to understand the potential steps I can take so I stop feeling lonely, factoring in

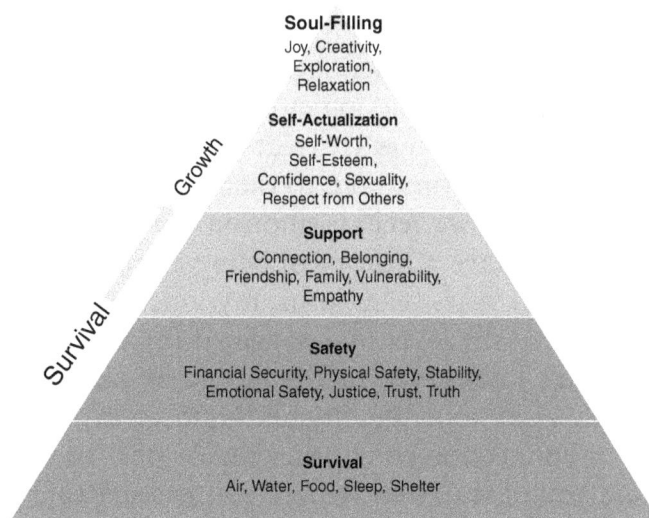

Figure 6.2 Hierarchy of Needs Chart

how well each step might work. Maybe my husband isn't feeling well, so I need to focus on adding connection with others in my life that day or week. That doesn't mean that connection with my husband isn't important in the long run, it means that we can balance out when we each have emotional bandwidth.

Making time for each other is important in any relationship, not just primary relationships, but balancing out what's going on for each person is just as important. It's part of identifying our limits, which we talked about earlier. For example, if I'm dealing with something difficult and want to talk through it with a good friend, but that friend is sick at the time, I'd need to either wait until they got better or talk with someone else if it was time sensitive. Considering the situation in a way that factors each person into the equation helps to ensure that needs are met for everyone.

Exercise 6–1:

1. Think of a recent time when you felt emotion or energy. Using the emotions chart, identify the core emotion and the specific emotions connected to that time.
2. What need was connected to that emotion?
3. What potential solutions might have met that need?

Balancing Triggers

Considering emotions and needs, recognize that including the past, present, and future is important. Our experiences are built as we go through life, so the emotions we feel often have historical context. "Triggers" are one of the better-known examples of how historical experiences impact emotion.

The term "trigger" is currently overused. It often is used to describe any strong emotion, or sometimes any emotion at all if you aren't used to feeling emotions. It actually refers to activation of our nervous system because something sends us the message that we are going to be harmed. This is often connected to a history of being harmed in a similar way. Triggered responses often appear to be stronger than the specific situation warrants. It's like opening a stuffed closet to try and put one more thing in it, but everything comes flying out because it's packed so tightly. Triggers are related to unresolved emotions, meaning we don't know how to meet the needs connected to them. Unresolved emotions are like links in a chain. Each experience where we feel an emotion that isn't resolved forms a link. If I feel lonely one afternoon, but I have a history of being abandoned throughout my life, or even throughout the last several years or months, my loneliness might feel much stronger. The loneliness might escalate to the level of a trigger if my experience with abandonment is strong enough that I doubt I am loved or I believe connection with others is not safe. If you've experienced betrayal in your life, in childhood, in a primary relationship or important relationship, or in connection to another major part of your life, often emotions like loneliness can remind you of situations where you weren't safe and didn't know if you could rely on others. Understanding the context of the trigger helps us understand how to meet the needs underneath and resolve the emotion.

As we discussed earlier, emotions aren't bad or good, they just give us information. If we translate that information, we can either make changes so we aren't hurting, or we can learn to do more of what we're doing because it makes us feel positive emotions. When a situation is resolved, we don't feel painful emotions in the same way. More significant pain requires more work to heal from, and some wounds change us forever, but peace and joy are possible no matter how much pain you've gone through.

As you move deeper into recovery, identifying your emotions and needs and the emotions and needs of those around you and balancing them is important. It can be difficult to determine how to find that balance. Often when there has been significant betrayal, one of two patterns emerge. Sometimes the person who betrayed feels they need to bend over backwards for the rest of their life to make it up to the person they hurt or make it up to the world in general. Sometimes the person who was betrayed feels like they need to walk on eggshells, or the other person will betray them again. Neither of these approaches is balanced.

Spending the rest of your life doing things you really don't want to do because you are scared of being betrayed again, or because you feel like you have to do it, isn't connective. That doesn't mean you ignore history. Context needs to be factored into the situation in a balanced way. If you hurt someone deeply, it's important to do what you can to support them as they heal and making sure you take the steps so you won't hurt them again. If it has long-term impacts, helping them deal with those impacts is important too. This isn't because you're bending over backwards. It's to honor the pain they've gone through.

For example, if you're riding a bike and do a trick you know is dangerous and you shouldn't be doing, and you crash and hit a friend and they break their arm, helping them as their arm heals is a good way to apologize. If the break causes them to struggle to take heavy boxes off high shelves in the future, then helping them take boxes down is way to continue to show them you care. Living your life constantly drowning in shame that you crashed into them and broke their arm isn't helpful. Being sensitive to short- and long-term costs to them is helpful.

Let's apply this to betrayal. Going through betrayal is often absolutely horrific. Hollenbeck and Steffens (2024) found that 84% of those who have gone through betrayal in their primary relationship felt anger stronger than anything else they've ever experienced, and two-thirds of them felt stuck in that anger. Understanding the depth of the pain experienced is essential for safe connection. We've already walked through steps you can take to understand that anger and pain and process through it. Helping someone you hurt through recovering from the pain caused by what you did is appropriate. Processing, recovery work, and time help to heal the pain. Therapeutic disclosure (in whatever format is best for you and your relationship) and changes to disconnecting and damaging relational dynamics also help.

As we move forward into middle recovery, awareness of the pain caused and empathy for potential continued impacts is vital. This cannot be at the expense of yourself, and it cannot be from a one-down position. Considering your own emotions and needs, along with understanding the emotions and needs of those connected to you, can help you work toward a more balanced approach.

Exercise 6–2:

1. Can you think of a time you were "triggered," meaning you had a very strong reaction to something that seemed stronger than might have initially made sense to you? What happened and what did you feel? Use the emotions chart and needs pyramid to figure out what emotions and needs were connected to the experience.
2. Thinking about that experience, what might it have been connected to from your past? When else have you experienced similar emotions?

Balanced Connection

Connection with self and others can be viewed as a balance between internal and external focus. As with many concepts, the idea of balance between the two can be understood when viewed as a continuum, with internal focus as one extreme and external focus as the other, and balanced connection in the middle. It might sound backwards, but the two ends of the continuum are at the expense of yourself. Neither end meets your needs or helps you connect in a healthy way with yourself and others. Whether you are internally focused or externally focused, the ends of the continuum are shame-based as you feel you don't have the right to exist and have healthy needs or healthy connection to others. The Balanced Connection Continuum diagram is available on the Connected Recovery® website if you'd like a visual representation of this material.

Significant internal focus concentrates on proving you are good enough to yourself. "Perfectionism" falls at this end of the continuum. Individuals with this mindset struggle to believe they are allowed to have human limits. They don't recognize their own needs and wants. Often this stems from unhealthy connection patterns in childhood, adolescence, or significant relationships. This is very much a dissociated state. If you think in terms of the emotional bucket we talked about in the introduction, individuals at this end of the continuum don't believe they have the right to have a bucket.

Most of us aren't the most extreme end of any continuum. Struggling with more mild internal focus imbalance might include struggles to trust others and a focus on being self-sufficient. Those at this point on the continuum might understand they have wants and needs, but they don't know how to ask for help or accept help if it's offered. Often they struggle with the belief that they have to do things on their own because they are the only ones who will do it correctly. This often stems from not being able to rely on others, but it's not quite as severe as those we described in the previous paragraph. It is a distant connection to others because others are kept at arm's length.

On the opposite end of the continuum, significant external focus, are those who look solely to others to try to prove to themselves that they are worthy of existing. They don't have boundaries and believe they are worth less than others, often believing they are broken beyond repair. Considering the emotional bucket, individuals on this end of the continuum have a bucket, but it's like there's no bottom to their bucket and they focus on having others continually pour water into the bucket, but the water goes straight through it. Unless there is a firehose on full blast, the bucket is empty. Because of this, they look for intensity rather than vulnerability and intimacy in connection because their need for connection is so severe that healthy, balanced interactions don't come close to meeting their needs.

A milder version of this might include struggling to have or maintain boundaries, in part because those leaning toward this side of the continuum believe their worth is based on the opinions of others. This level of connection is enmeshed because happiness, safety, and success are in the hands of others, which makes it difficult to feel at peace.

When considering where you might fall on this continuum, recognize that usually it's more of a pendulum. Sometimes we might be rusted into place on one side or another, but usually we swing back and forth between internally focused and externally focused, especially as we do the work to see ourselves and our patterns more clearly. If we see our patterns as a ball on the end of a rope that swings back and forth between each side, our goal is to shorten the rope and move closer to the middle. We're human, so we will never be exactly in the middle, but as we process through our patterns and learn to find a balance between advocating for ourselves and factoring in empathy for others, we shorten the rope. See Figure 6.3. A full-sized version of this diagram is available on ConnectedRecoveryTraining.com.

The middle of this continuum is balanced connection. Balanced connection allows us to have healthy boundaries that protect us while maximizing our connection to others. It incorporates self-compassion and empathy for those around us. It allows us to accept ourselves and others because we have the skills to create safety for ourselves and within our relationships. Those at this point on the continuum have built reliable and safe connections with themselves and others. They have learned how to ask for help when needed, and they have connections in their life that offer help in balanced ways. Additionally, they can offer help to others in a way that honors their own limits and respects the limits of others. They recognize that they have the right to say no to even reasonable requests.

Remember, anytime someone asks something of us, we always have the right to consider what response best fits us. This applies whether or not the request is phrased as a request. An expectation is a request. A demand is a request. When someone makes a request, we have three choices. We can say "yes, I can do that," "no, I can't do that," or "I can't do that, but I can offer this instead." While we have the ability to choose whether or not

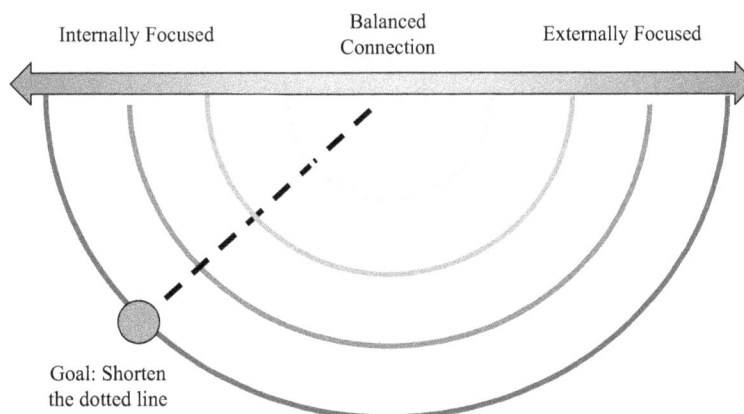

Internally Focused   Balanced   Externally Focused
                           Connection

Goal: Shorten
the dotted line

Figure 6.3 Balanced Continuum Pendulum Diagram

we want to do something, we can't pick how someone responds to it or change how our choice impacts the situation. For example, if you get in a fight with a significant other, they might want to talk through what happened. You can choose to talk to them, choose not to talk to them, or offer another option, such as, "This feels like both of us have a lot of energy connected to the situation. Could we talk about this in our next therapy session?" If you choose not to talk through it with them or offer another way to resolve the situation, there will likely be more distance in your relationship with them and the way you connect with them might change.

Tying this information to the first half of this chapter, understanding our emotions and needs and recognizing the emotions and needs of others can help us determine what requests we want to make to others and how to respond to requests others make to us. This balance helps us to create a deeper and safer connection to ourselves and others.

Exercise 6–3:

1. Where do you currently see yourself on the Balanced Connection Continuum? Do you tend to lean more toward internal focus, external focus, or somewhere in between?
2. What steps might be helpful to work toward balanced connection, where you both advocate for yourself and consider the needs of others?

Super Short Summary:

Emotions aren't bad or good. They give us information. Needs are general; they aren't the solutions to meet our needs, rather they help us identify potential solutions. Triggers are strong emotional reactions that activate our nervous systems and are related to unresolved emotions we've experienced throughout life. Healthy connection is balanced connection, where individuals honor their needs while maintaining empathy and appropriate boundaries with others. Recognizing emotional patterns, understanding triggers, and learning to balance personal needs with those of others helps build deeper, healthier connections.

Chapter Questions:

1. What did you connect to the most in this chapter?
2. What steps are you taking to apply this material to your life?
3. How can you use what you've learned in this chapter to create deeper, more meaningful connections in your life?

7

Honesty

Attachment and Family of Origin

The honesty component of middle recovery focuses on attachment and family-of-origin work. To dig deeper into understanding ourselves, we need to consider where we came from and how it impacted us and our ability to connect to ourselves and others. We need to identify and heal any wounds that were created.

Attachment

John Bowlby, an English psychiatrist and psychoanalyst, spent his career considering how humans are impacted by the connection they have with others, starting at birth. He developed a model called Attachment Theory (1982). Attachment Theory explains that connection to others is a biological need and that our experiences shape the way we connect with others. Secure attachment means we can trust ourselves and others. Insecure attachment means we have learned that we can't feel safe in our connection with self and others.

Bartholomew and Horowitz (1991) created a graph that divided attachment styles into four categories. The four categories were defined based on two concepts – anxiety and avoidance. Anxiety considered fear of rejection or abandonment, and avoidance looked at discomfort with closeness. The chart they created looked like a graph with anxiety stretching from right (low anxiety) to left (high anxiety), and avoidance stretching from top (low avoidance) to bottom (high avoidance). This chart is still used to measure attachment style.

The upper left-hand square of the diagram includes low anxiety and low avoidance, which indicates secure attachment. The upper right-hand square, including high anxiety and low avoidance, is labeled anxious attachment. Low anxiety and high avoidance, the bottom left-hand square, indicates avoidant attachment. The remaining square, which includes high avoidance and high anxiety, is now known as disorganized attachment. Historically, it was called anxious-avoidant attachment or fearful-avoidant attachment.

A study done by Mary Ainsworth and colleagues (1978) helped to define the first three attachment styles. Her study focused on mothers and toddlers. She had the mothers bring their young children into a playroom, leave for a bit, and then return. She watched how the toddlers responded to each part of the process. Personally, as a mother of six, I know that some of how we respond is based on personality, but Ainsworth's study gives a good foundation to understand what different types of attachment mean. Children with secure attachment wanted their mother there, missed them when they left, but were easily

DOI: 10.4324/9781003623359-10

comforted when the mom returned. This showed that they knew their mother would meet their needs and provide a safe environment for them. Those with anxious attachment were very upset when their mother left and continued to be upset at them after they returned. Basically, this translates to believing that their mother might meet their needs but not knowing if they would or not, so they continually are wondering if they are going to be taken care of or not. Children with the third attachment style, avoidant attachment, barely noticed when their mom left and when they returned. This type of attachment style indicates that they don't believe others will meet their needs, so they just take care of themselves.

The fourth attachment style, disorganized attachment, was not added until eight years later by Main and Solomon (1986). Disorganized attachment is created when the person you rely on is both the source of your pain and the person you look to for comfort and safety. The individual doesn't know what to do and often goes back and forth between trying to connect and pulling away. This style of attachment comes from severe trauma or abuse. Attachment wounds created by betrayal often create reactions that are similar to those seen in children with disorganized attachment (Rokach & Chan, 2023; Warach & Josephs, 2021) because in both cases, the pain was caused by someone who was trusted and relied on to create safety, often someone they long to be connected with.

While our experiences in infancy and childhood have been shown to have a strong impact on the way we view connection as we go through life, our connections in adulthood can shape how safe we feel with ourselves and others. It's also important to realize that we can heal from our attachment wounds, and it is possible to shift into a secure attachment style (Fraley et al., 2021).

Exercise 7–1:

1. Consider your connection with others. Do you feel more anxiety or more avoidance? Or do you feel secure?
2. How has the way you connect with others changed throughout your life?

Family-of-Origin Dynamics

Let's talk more about family dynamics. Please note that the term "family" applies to the individuals you were primarily connected to. In this section, we're going to learn about Adverse Childhood Experiences (ACEs), family rules, and family roles. Each one may have pieces of the puzzle that help you understand yourself and those connected to you better. As with any topic, some of this might not apply to you, but exploring these areas often helps us to better understand the patterns each of us has.

As we discuss this topic, it may be difficult to consider the dysfunctional patterns in your family-of-origin. Our goal is to identify and understand those patterns so you can shift into healthier patterns. We aren't trying to convince you that your family members were bad; we're looking at the patterns to give you a chance to see harmful patterns or pain you've experienced, so you can better heal from them. There absolutely are family systems that cause significant damage to the children connected to them and strict boundaries are necessary in those cases. While families like that exist, most dysfunctional families love each other but lack the skills or tools to change generational patterns. They weren't taught any other way to interact. These steps teach you how to see some of those patterns, so you can be more connected with yourself and with others. If your family members were the ones going through this process, we'd ask them to consider the same questions and concepts. Disconnecting patterns are taught and developed because of pain, but they also cause pain. We're working to change those patterns so you and those connected with you feel less pain and more joy and peace.

ACEs

In Chapter 1 we learned about trauma cycles. The foundations behind our trauma cycle responses in adulthood are often formed in childhood. Understanding trauma we experienced in childhood can help us identify targets to process through in recovery. One tool to help identify traumatic experiences in childhood is ACEs, which stands for Adverse Childhood Experiences. The ACE study (Felitti et al., 1998) determined that trauma we experience in the first 18 years of our life can have long-term impacts on us.

The ACE study divided childhood trauma into two general categories: abuse and household dysfunction. Research around ACEs has been ongoing and later research added neglect as a third category (CDC, 2016a). The abuse category covered physical, emotional, and sexual abuse. Household dysfunction explored substance abuse by anyone in the household, parental separation or divorce, domestic violence, having a member of the household struggle with mental illness, or having a family member incarcerated. The neglect category considered physical and emotional neglect.

As we discussed when we talked about attachment, healing is possible, even if you've experienced significant trauma. When we go through something significant enough to make us believe our world isn't safe, it creates data points in our heads and hearts that can make it difficult to rebuild trust. This is the same concept we talked about much earlier in this book when we discussed what betrayal trauma is. As Herman (1992) explained, the "trauma" part of betrayal trauma comes from not knowing if you will ever be able to protect yourself from being hurt in the same way again. Experiences that show us our world and our connections are safe give us alternate data points and help us to heal. Those types of experiences might include supportive relationships, safe environments, or resources (CDC, 2016b).

Family Rules

Models of therapy that focus on family systems (Bowen, 1978; Minuchin, 1974; Satir, 1964) state that every family, just like every organization and every relationship of any type, has rules. Sometimes some of those rules are written down, for example in a business contract, company, or religion. Usually, families don't write their rules down. Sometimes the family rules aren't even stated overtly, they are just understood by everyone. They define how you should behave, communicate, and interact with others, both those within the family system and those outside of the family system. They are shared expectations and boundaries (not necessarily healthy boundaries) for the family system as a whole.

Families that function in an unhealthy way tend to have three basic rules – don't talk, don't feel, and don't question. Don't talk often means don't talk about the things you don't like, along with don't tell anyone else what happens in the family. Don't feel is usually covertly conveyed by shutting family members down if they try to express emotions. It may also be overtly conveyed by phrases such as "Don't cry or I'll give you something to cry about." Don't question stops family members from challenging decisions made. "Because I said so" is an overt way to state this rule. As with the other two rules, it is also often conveyed covertly, in this case by shutting down anyone who tries to change the way things are handled. All three rules often prevent family members from identifying dysfunction within the family, processing through pain caused by the dysfunction, and changing the patterns.

Omar Minwalla (2021) discusses a concept that can give helpful context for understanding family patterns that may have helped to build unhealthy patterns of communication. He states that those who struggle with patterns of problematic sexual behaviors often have a "secret sexual basement," meaning they have aspects of themselves they feel significant shame around and deliberately hide from others, and sometimes even from themselves. There are two aspects of this that I feel are vital and apply to everyone, not just those who are struggling with problematic sexual behaviors. The first question I ask if I have someone come into my office who says that they read his material and connected to the idea of a secret sexual basement is "who taught you to build a basement?" The second essential consideration is that "secret basements" aren't just sexual. There are multiple aspects of ourselves that we may have been taught to hide. Cleaning out those secret basements, whatever happens to be in them, is a critical step to feeling connection to ourselves and making connection with others safe.

All three family rules help to build secret basements. "Don't talk" stops you from talking about problems, emotions, or personal experiences. Family members are taught to keep quiet about difficult topics such as escape patterns, abuse, or even financial struggles. Secrets are kept to maintain the façade of being a "normal family" and to avoid conflict within the family system. Conversation focuses on surface-level topics and anyone who tries to bring up deeper topics is punished, rejected, or made fun of. Phrases that align with this rule include "it's not a big deal" and "we don't need to talk about that."

"Don't feel" teaches you to suppress or ignore your emotions, possibly even learning to deny they exist. This especially applies to painful emotions like anger, sadness, or fear. In dysfunctional families, emotions are often viewed as a sign of weakness. Emotionless functioning is viewed as being strong. Rationality and productivity are prioritized over emotional well-being. This rule teaches children to suppress their emotions to "support" the family, often at the expense of their developmental needs. Common phrases connected to this rule are "you're too sensitive" and "just get over it and move on."

The third rule, "don't question" teaches blind obedience to authority. Others are not allowed to question the rationale behind or fairness of decisions and actions. Power dynamics are rigid. This structure prevents those in power from being held accountable for their actions and allows abusive or harmful behaviors to be ignored or justified. Anyone who questions the family dynamics is seen as disloyal or rebellious.

I love the quote made popular by Patsy Clairmont (1998): "Normal is just a setting on a dryer." There is no such thing as normal. Every family has some level of dysfunction because families are made up of human beings. A larger percentage of families than you would guess has a high level of dysfunction, we just don't see it, so we shame ourselves and think we are more broken than others. Especially in today's world where our experiences are conveyed largely through social media, we don't see an accurate picture of others. Most people don't post dysfunction on social media, you only see the good parts of what's going on with them. Someone commented on a social media post I made about this topic (yes, I recognize it's ironic to use a reference to a social media post in this paragraph) that all we see is their "highlight reel." Understanding this can help normalize seeing dysfunction, allowing us to process through it and change our patterns.

Changing these rules for ourselves and within the systems we are connected to helps to heal the pain caused by the dysfunction and prevents the painful patterns from continuing. To break these rules, start with encouraging conversation. Do the emotional work you need to do to show up for difficult conversations and stay grounded. Process through your experiences so you can understand how they impacted you and you can share them when it's appropriate and emotionally safe. Recognize that emotions are important, even if they are painful. Work to identify and share your emotions in a grounded way. Healthy emotional expression allows you to work through conflict. Incorporate mutual respect as part of conversations. Give yourself and others permission to challenge ideas or behaviors, considering if they are healthy patterns. Seek help when you need it. Deeper conversations provide an opportunity for growth, connection, and healing.

Recognize that you likely will not be able to make significant changes to your family-of-origin unless the majority of your family members are willing to work toward those changes, which doesn't happen very often. Often the only steps we can take with the families we grew up in are identifying the dysfunctional patterns and setting boundaries for ourselves that minimize the impact those patterns can have on us. As we talked about in Chapter 3, this actually maximizes the connection we have with them. If we set healthy boundaries for ourselves, we minimize their ability to hurt us, so we can spend more time with them and the time we spend with them is more connecting. This isn't about blame, it's about safety, healing, and connection.

Exercise 7–2:

1. What were some of the rules in your family when you were growing up?
2. Have you brought any of those rules into your current family? If so, which ones?
3. Are there any rules from your family-of-origin that you have actively worked to change in your current family dynamics? If so, what are they?
4. Do you think your family has any secret basements? Do you have any secret basements? If so, what is in them?
5. Did this section bring up painful thoughts or realizations for you? If so, process through those with your therapist or support system.

Family Roles

Family system models of therapy (Bowen, 1978; Minuchin, 1974; Satir, 1964) also agree that there are different roles within each family system. Several of these roles were initially defined through exploring dynamics related to families that included individuals struggling with alcoholism (Black, 1982; Wegscheider-Cruse, 1981), which would fall into escape cycles like those we discussed in Chapter 1.

Four roles that were explained by Black (1982) and Wegscheider-Cruse (1981) are: hero, scapegoat, mascot, and lost child. I've also found it helpful to consider the following roles: golden child (Wegscheider-Cruse, 1981), black sheep (Wegscheider-Cruse, 1981), and caretaker (Black, 1982; Satir, 1964). Let's explore each of these. As you read through them, consider which ones you connect to and which ones you see in your family-of-origin dynamics.

The hero role applies to the "perfect" family member. They make the family and the parental figures look good. This is often an attempt by the family system to distract from or compensate for dysfunction in the family. Those placed in the role of hero often feel they aren't allowed to fail. They may struggle with anxiety and perfectionism. This role teaches you that you have to be perfect, that you have to continually work to earn your right to be part of the system, and that you aren't allowed to have limits.

The scapegoat on the other hand, is the one who is blamed for all the problems in the family. This is also often an attempt to distract from the dysfunctional patterns. Individuals placed in the scapegoat role often believe they really are the problem. They might struggle with internalized shame, the belief that there is something inherently wrong with them and they are defective.

The mascot of the family is the class clown. Their job is to relieve tension and distract others from family problems. This is a more generalized version of the "shield" response in the list of survival responses. Living in this role can make you feel like your only response to painful patterns is humor. It can make it difficult to believe you can express your emotions and be taken seriously.

The lost child is the invisible member of the family. They stay quiet because they have been taught they aren't allowed to ask others for attention, connection, or emotional energy. They often become very independent and isolated. Those in this role may struggle to form close relationships because they have been taught they aren't supposed to be seen.

The golden child role is similar to the hero role. The primary difference is that the golden child can do no wrong. They may not actually be a high achiever, but they are viewed as one. This role teaches them that they will never have consequences for what they do. It can lead to feeling entitled.

The black sheep role is a variation of the scapegoat role. While the scapegoat believes they are the problem, the black sheep often refuses to follow the family dysfunctional patterns and may be outcast for their refusal to play the game and live by the disconnecting family rules. Other family members will blame the black sheep for any problems in the family as a way to divert attention from deeper family issues.

The caretaker role was initially explained by Satir (1964) and expounded on by Black (1982). Similar to the mascot, the caretaker's job is to keep the family stable and balance out the dysfunction. While mascots distract to maintain the status quo, caretakers are often expected to predict and meet the needs of others, controlling the impact emotions have on others, at the expense of their own needs.

Every family system is different. If you were raised in multiple systems, for example if your parental figures lived separately or got divorced, you may have played different roles in each part of your system. Family roles are created to survive in a dysfunctional system. As children, we don't have the option to opt out of the system, and we have very little power to change it. Understanding the roles we step into helps us to better connect to ourselves and others because we are able to internally shift out of the roles and determine how we want to interact moving forward.

Even if the changes you make are very healthy, often systems don't change with us. Systems actually do the opposite. They work to stay the same. Don't be surprised if your family strongly disagrees with your conclusions regarding the work you do to identify unhealthy and disconnecting patterns. You might need to set up new boundaries and build new connections as you move forward.

Exercise 7–3:

1. What family roles did you connect with? Why?
2. What roles might other family members have filled?
3. How have the roles in your family-of-origin impacted your connection with yourself and others?

Super Short Summary:

Our attachment style relates to how we connect with others and is measured by considering our level of anxiety in relation to connection with others versus our level of avoidance. Our attachment style is developed in childhood but can be strongly influenced by our relationships throughout our lives. Childhood trauma can be measured using the ACEs scale. Dysfunctional families often have three rules: don't talk, don't feel, and don't question. Dysfunctional families also often put family members in specific roles, such as scapegoat, mascot, or caregiver. Understanding those rules and roles can help us change the patterns.

Chapter Questions:

1. What did you connect to the most in this chapter?
2. What steps are you taking to apply this material to your life?

8

Boundaries

Relational Patterns and Boundaries

Now that we understand emotions and needs better and have explored attachment styles and family-of-origin dynamics, let's expand on the last question you answered in Chapter 7 – how do the disconnecting patterns from our past influence current relational patterns and what steps might be helpful to change those dynamics? This question helps us explore the third component of the Connected Recovery® model, boundaries, as it relates to middle recovery.

Relational Pattern Tools

Multiple practitioners have developed tools to see relational patterns more clearly. Different approaches often give us different insights about ourselves and the behaviors and reactions that apply to us. Let's explore a few tools that help identify relational patterns.

Identifying Relational Patterns

Dr. Sue Johnson (2004, 2008) created a model of relational therapy called emotionally focused therapy (EFT). This model is founded in Attachment Theory, which we talked about in the last chapter. It focuses on the relational patterns, which Johnson calls "dances" because we tend to repeat the same steps each time we have conflict. While the original model was created for couples, it applies to all human relationships. EFT has been shown to apply cross-culturally (Allan et al., 2022; Nightingale et al., 2019) and across relational orientation, meaning it is helpful for relationships other than monogamous connections (Edwards et al., 2023).

If you have a long-term connection with someone, have you noticed that you often repeat the same fights? The details might differ, but the arguments likely follow the same pattern. These are our "dances." Addressing context only allows us to find resolution for a specific situation. Considering the patterns we use to communicate allows us to change those patterns, giving us the chance to incorporate tools that help us to better deal with conflict.

The first step to changing our patterns is to identify them and understand what drives them. This is done by considering the pattern, then looking at the emotions and needs underneath the behaviors and finally shifting into working together with the other or others involved in the pattern to see the pattern as the issue rather than seeing each other as the problem.

DOI: 10.4324/9781003623359-11

Johnson (2004, 2008) describes three specific dances. If you connect to this material, she wrote *Hold Me Tight* (2008) to walk people through EFT and how it applies to them. It provides much more detail than what I'll summarize below. The three dances explore the three possible combinations based on responses falling into two categories – pursue or withdraw. Pursuers believe that working through the issue in the moment is absolutely needed, no matter what collateral damage ensues, while withdrawers shut off because they are overwhelmed. Pursuers continue to push for the situation to be addressed despite the damage the conversation is causing, and withdrawers try to leave the conversation and brush it under the rug.

The first dance Johnson details is the "protest polka." This is a combination of at least one pursuer and at least one withdrawer. Each person feels hurt as the pursuers feel rejected and the withdrawers feel overwhelmed or inadequate. The second dance is "freeze and flee." In this case, each person in the equation withdraws and shuts down. Conflict is never resolved because it is minimized and avoided. The third is "find the bad guy" and each party is a pursuer. This dance focuses on blame and criticism, escalating and causing significant collateral damage.

Exercise 8–1:

1. Are you a pursuer or withdrawer? Or do you play different roles depending on who you're connected to?
2. Consider those you've been or are currently in a primary relationship with. Are they pursuers or withdrawers?
3. Which of the dances have you experienced in the various connections you've had with others?

Hula Hoops

Mark and Debbie Laaser (2017) created an exercise they call "The Hoops." I've found their imaging of the three hoops (or however many you need to illustrate the relationship you're focusing on in the exercise – you'll need one hoop for each person and one hoop signifying the relationship) very helpful. They sell a PDF booklet on their website (faithfulandtrue.com) that describes how they use the exercise in detail with photos. While I use slightly different language (they explain it as stages of relationship development), the concepts I use with clients are very similar to those they explain in their booklet. This tool can be used to map a primary relationship, a family's dynamic, or even connection between friends.

This is an experiential (meaning not just talk therapy) exercise related to psychodrama, a modality of therapy where you use action to represent what you feel. I use this imagery enough that I have a set of hula hoops in the corner of my office. When I use them with clients, I pull out one for each individual in the relationship and one representing the relationship. My default set up is to have each individual hula hoop touch the relational hula hoop. I've found it helpful to let clients adjust the position of their individual hula hoops as a visual representation of their current level of connection. Sometimes all hoops are close together. Other times the individual hoops are as far apart as possible.

Each individual's hoop represents their own beliefs and values, their experiences, their recovery (whatever that means for each person), their emotions, and their needs. The relational hoop represents bids for connection and mutual interdependency. This visualization helps to illustrate your own view of the situation and to identify when you're considering your own emotions and needs versus when you are numbing and stepping away from the relationship, or when you are trying to see everyone else's emotions and needs and change their behaviors.

Often, I'll have clients use the hoops as they work through a conflict. When explaining what happened, if they shift into saying what someone else thought or did, I have them step into that person's hoop. It's interesting to watch reactions when that happens. How comfortable would you be if someone stepped into your hoop? Most people are very uncomfortable having someone in their space, so they respond by working to change the situation. Sometimes they step out of their hoop. Other times they push the other person out of their hoop. If the person steps out of their hoop, I might ask how that feels to the individual who is now standing in another individual's hoop. Then I ask them who is in their hoop – no one is. No one is advocating for them or showing up for them. I will also ask the person who has stepped away, out of their hoop, how they feel. I'll have them consider what it's like to have someone else in their hoop and what it's like to step away from the relationship.

Applying the concepts we discussed in Chapter 1, escape cycles often involve stepping out of our hula hoop and away from connection. Trauma cycles might involve stepping away (flight, freeze, or fold), stepping out of our hoop trying to manage someone else, or everyone else's hoop (fawn or frenzy), or increasing the energy in our response (fight). Considering the EFT dances, pursuers tend to step in other people's hoops and withdrawers tend to step out of the hoops.

Healthy connection does not involve leaving our hula hoop or stepping into someone else's. We keep one foot in our hoop and put one foot in the relational hoop, offering the chance for others to put one foot in the relational hoop and work together with us to process through experiences, work through conflict, and share pieces of our lives. By keeping one foot in our hoop, we make sure we stay aware of all the data points, including our emotions and needs. We make sure we are advocated for. We also offer bids for connection but offer it from a grounded place.

Exercise 8–2:

1. Consider the important relationships in your life. What do you think the hula hoop arrangement would look like?
2. Do you think you are more likely to step in someone else's hoop or step out of the equation? What does that response give you?
3. What would you need to work on to better understand your own hula hoop?
4. What steps might be helpful to make the relational hoop safer for you?

Relational Compass

We talked in Chapter 2 about creating a personal compass using Dr. Caudill's exercise. This can be a helpful relational tool as well. There may be similarities between your personal compass and your relational compass, but understanding the differences can be helpful. They could also be completely different. Let's consider the different parts of the compass exercise in the context of your work to connect with others, whether that's within your primary relationship, your family relationships, or in relationships in general. Pick one to focus on as you're reading this part of the book. You can always go back and focus on a different relationship later if needed. Pull out something to write on.

What are you working toward in that relationship? What is your north for that relationship? This could be long-term or short-term. It could be an emotional goal or something that's happening. For example, if one of you is working on a degree, a short-term goal could be focusing on finishing school. You could also choose to focus on what you want to build in the relationship long-term. For example, with my children, my long-term goal with them is connection. I want to have a strong relationship with them as they get older.

What drives you in this relationship? What is pushing you forward? This would be south on your diagram. Considering the example above, if you're working toward finishing school, perhaps financial stability or flexibility in the options you'll have in the future might be driving you. If you're considering a primary relationship, longevity or love might drive you.

What redirects you toward your north? Pick two as this is east and west on the diagram. In the example of working toward a degree, one of these might be continued reevaluation. If you struggle to wonder if it's worth it, reviewing the situation might be helpful to keep you moving forward. Another option for this position might be support. When I was working to finish my PhD, I had two friends specifically who wouldn't let me quit. They refused to let me believe I couldn't do it, and when I faltered, they made me figure out my next step forward. There's no way I would have made it without them. Different things drive different people and relationships. Considering my long-term friendships, making sure I spend time with them might be important for either east or west.

In the middle of your relational compass, put what centers you for this relationship. What keeps you grounded? What anchors you? This is the foundation. It's what matters most to you. It's the truth that keeps you steady. If I had created a compass around getting my PhD, I would have put "street cred" in the middle. One of my kiddos asked me why I was getting the degree. I explained to them that I needed to have a PhD because I was teaching individuals with master's and doctoral level degrees. They responded with "so basically it's for street cred?" Yes. Street cred. It made us laugh, but it represented increased job security. It represented increased ability to reach others and provide tools that would help heal pain. My husband, my kiddos, and I worked toward my degree for those reasons.

Exercise 8–3:

1. What came up for you as you created your relational compass?
2. How might you use this moving forward with that relationship?
3. What other relationships might it be helpful for you to create a relational compass for?

Relational Three Circles

We talked about the three circles in Chapter 3. The version of the three circles that applies to middle recovery I call the relational three circles. A diagram of this is available at ConnectedRecoveryTraining.com if you'd like a visual. As we understand more about ourselves and the way we interact with others, we can use the relational three circles to organize different actions or reactions. The relational three circles considers if behaviors are connecting, disconnecting, or damaging. It can be helpful to use what you've learned about yourself from the previous exercises in this chapter (and potentially what you've learned about yourself in other chapters). The relational compass can help determine which category behaviors fall into as well. Do they help you move toward north on your relational compass? Each person and each relationship will have different behaviors that fall into each category. As with bucket-fillers in the introduction, what's connecting for one person might be disconnecting or even damaging for another.

Connecting behaviors actively nurture and strengthen your connection to others, while also strengthening your connection to yourself. These behaviors strengthen your emotional bonds and build trust. Behaviors in this category might include identifying your limits and communicating them, active listening, making time for check-ins and connection at some level each day, and setting up dates. The term "dates" can apply to any relationship – I go on dates with my husband, take my kids on "mommy dates," go out with friends for girls' nights out or a friends' night out, go on double dates with others in relationships, and go out with my husband and one of my best friends. Working through conflict might be on your list of connecting behaviors and it's important to consider what steps have worked well for you to resolve conflict within that relationship.

Disconnecting behaviors unintentionally create emotional distance or prevent connection. These behaviors often stem from stress, lack of awareness, or skills you need to develop but haven't worked on yet. As with other definitions, these will differ by person and relationship. Regarding this tool specifically, what falls into disconnecting behaviors as opposed to damaging behaviors will differ depending on personal triggers and pain points, relational history, and individual history. For example, some people might list "ignoring irritations" as a disconnecting behavior, but if you have a history of ignoring small irritations, building resentment, and using resentment as an excuse to deceive or betray, it might be more important to focus on verbalizing irritations, even if they are small. Just as we discussed in Chapter 3, this part of your three circles diagram can include items that you don't have control over and items you have more control over, but don't quite fall into the category of damaging behaviors. For example, perhaps one of you going on business trips makes it more difficult to connect. That doesn't mean going on business trips is damaging, it means you'll need to be aware that they increase disconnection. By putting it on your list of disconnecting behaviors, you can increase your awareness of it.

The third category, which is the center of your three circles on the diagram, is relationally damaging behaviors. This category includes behaviors you absolutely want to avoid because they erode trust and safety, deepen conflict, and can lead to significant relational problems. These will differ by person and by relationship. Criticism or contempt might be on this list, along with invalidating a partner's feelings. Using threats or coercion might be included. Dishonesty might be on the list as well. It may be helpful to consider levels of different behaviors, and the behaviors might belong in different categories based on the severity.

I recommend you review the behaviors in the last two categories and consider why you have done them in the past. What goal were you trying to work toward? Then consider if there is a more effective, grounded, and connecting way to work toward that goal. For example, criticism might have been used in the past to try and address a partner's patterns or behaviors that cause you pain. Consider how you could communicate about these issues in a healthier way. Don't just try to avoid doing behaviors you've done in the past. It's like going on a diet – not only do you need to work on not eating unhealthy foods, but you need to add healthy foods.

Exercise 8–4:

1. What behaviors and activities might you include in the outer circle of your relational three circles (connecting behaviors)?
2. What behaviors and actions might fit best in the second part of your three circles (disconnecting behaviors)?
3. What might fit in the center of your relational three circles (damaging behaviors)?
4. Consider your answers from questions 2 and 3. Why were you using those behaviors? What might you replace them with? Which ones would it be helpful to discuss with your therapist or support system to get help working on alternative approaches?

Relational Boundaries

We talked about boundaries in Chapter 3. Each phase of the Connected Recovery® model deepens the work we've done in the previous phases. With the tools we've covered in the last chapter, and what you've learned about yourself since Chapter 3, consider how this information changes the boundaries you have for your connection to yourself and your connection with others.

As we discussed earlier, boundaries protect and connect. When we know where our limits are and we have the ability to protect ourselves from being pushed beyond our limits, we maximize our ability to connect with ourselves and others. Let's review what we've covered in this phase of recovery and how it might impact our boundaries. As you go through this section, write your answers down.

How have you and those connected to you been impacted by behaviors and patterns in the past? As you consider that question, explore what support you or they might need and how that can be provided in a balanced way. What boundaries do you need as you move forward that acknowledge the pain, but don't create a power imbalance?

Review what you learned about yourself and how balanced your connection is between being internally focused versus externally focused. What boundaries might be helpful for you to become more balanced? It's ok to return to that part of the book (Chapter 6) to consider what steps might be helpful.

Considering your attachment style, and perhaps how you perceive the attachment style of those connected to you, what boundaries would help to build a world where you are safe to explore? Where you can rely on yourself and others in your life? What boundaries can help you move toward more secure attachment?

Along a similar vein, consider the role you filled in your family-of-origin. What might you need to be able to step out of the role? What boundaries and actions would be helpful as you take those steps? Also consider the rules you had in your family-of-origin and the rules that exist in your current relationships. What boundaries do you need to set up for yourself and those connected to you to help shift those rules into healthier patterns? What secrets are in your secret basements and what boundaries might help you make sure those basements get cleaned out?

When we discussed EFT and the different relational conflict patterns, did you connect more as a pursuer or a withdrawer? What patterns did you identify in your relational conflicts? What boundaries might be helpful to change those patterns? Also consider what your hula hoop structure might look like. What boundaries might be helpful for you to stay in your hula hoop, keep others out of your hoop, and allow you to put a foot into your relational hoop when desired?

Finally consider your relational three circles. What boundaries do you need to set up for yourself and within your relationships to help identify when disconnecting and damaging behaviors show up? How would you like to respond when they do?

Exercise 8–5:

1. Review the answers you've written down. Combine them into a list of boundaries you would like to set up for yourself and your relationships.
2. Consider your list and determine which areas might be helpful to review with your therapist or support system? Are there any you need help with?
3. Are there any relational boundaries that might be helpful to discuss with others in the relationship? If so, what steps could you take to do so?

Super Short Summary:

Often our disconnection with others follows general patterns. Identifying the general patterns our disconnection follows allows us to change those patterns. An important part of relational patterns is knowing how to advocate for yourself and recognizing the boundaries you need, while balancing self-advocation with empathy for and awareness of others.

Chapter Questions:

1. What did you connect to the most in this chapter?
2. What steps are you taking to apply this material to your life?

Chapter 9

Communication

Purposeful Sharing

Deeper understanding of yourself, the patterns you've seen and developed throughout your life, and the relational boundaries you need all help to create a foundation where you can share more vulnerably. We address this in the communication component of middle recovery. This includes two aspects – how much you want to share and how you want to share it.

Interpersonal Transparency

Interpersonal transparency refers to how much we want to share, how open we want to be with someone else. It also includes how much we want to let in from others – are we interested in hearing what they think about us and what they see in us? Recognize that we need to feel safe with someone to be interested in listening to their thoughts about us. This concept applies to any connection, including primary relationships, family relationships, friendships, and professional relationships.

Johari's Window is a model created in 1955 by Joseph Luft and Harrington Ingham that explains interpersonal communication and self-awareness, which are the two parts of interpersonal transparency. Luft and Ingham's model divided information based on two elements, known to self and known to others. Their diagram for this concept included four squares – open (known to self and others), blind (known to others, but not seen by self), hidden (known to self, but not shared with others), and unknown (not known to self or seen by others).

As Luft and Ingham illustrated, interpersonal connection includes two elements; how we understand ourselves and how others see us. I view those two aspects as a Venn diagram, which is two circles that are overlapping (see Figure 9.1). In this situation, one circle is what we know and understand about ourselves and the conclusions we've drawn from that information (self-awareness). The other circle is what others see about us and the conclusions they've drawn from that information (assumptions). Keep in mind that some aspects of both circles will be accurate, some will be partially accurate, and some will be inaccurate. The work we do to understand ourselves and the experiences we've gone through increase our self-awareness and therefore make that circle more accurate. The more work others have done on themselves and the experiences they've gone through, the more accurate their assumptions about us will be. The area where the two circles overlap

DOI: 10.4324/9781003623359-12

Level 1
Meaningful Contacts
(150)

Level 2
Friends
(up to 50)

Known to Self Shared Seen or Assumed by Others

Level 3
Good Friends
(up to 15)

Level 4
Close Friends
(up to 5)

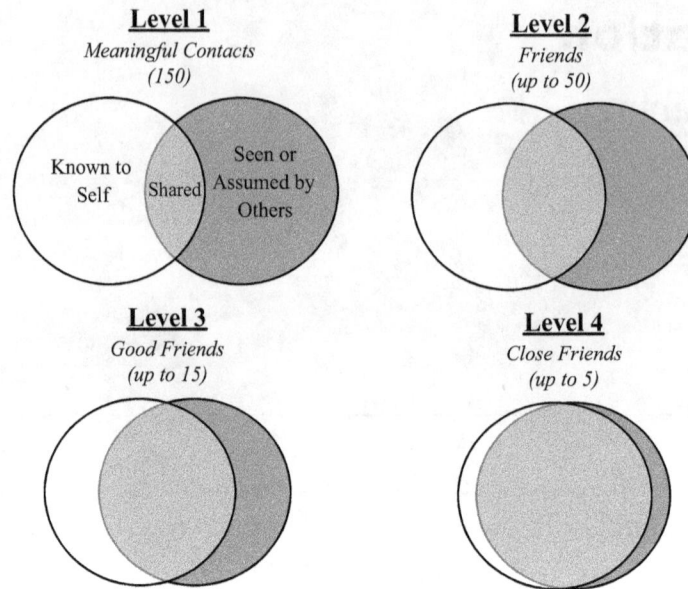

Figure 9.1 Relationship Levels Diagram

represents what is shared, both about what we know about ourselves and what others see in us. The more the circles overlap, the closer the relationship is.

Boundaries help us figure out how much we want to share with others and how much we want to accept feedback from them. Sharing without boundaries leads to pain, although not sharing at all leads to a different type of pain – loneliness and isolation. Healthy connection provides a space where each individual can be open and authentic, and each person is seen and valued. The depth of interpersonal transparency is determined by the depth of the connection, trust, understanding, and safety in a relationship.

We have a limited amount of time, energy, and emotional bandwidth. Because of this, our ability to connect to others at deeper levels is limited. Robin Dunbar, an anthropologist and evolutionary psychologist, created a concept that explains the different levels of social connection. This is called Dunbar's Number (1992, 1998). He divided the different levels of social connection into four layers: intimate friends, good friends, friends, and meaningful contacts. His studies determined that we can maintain at most five close friendships, 15 good friendships, 50 general friendships, and 150 meaningful contacts (1998). See Figure 9.1 for a visual representation of how interpersonal transparency looks at different relationship levels.

In my experience, everyone needs connections at each of these levels, although you may not need the maximum number at each level. Different people will need different amounts of connection. While you may not need or want 15 good friends and five close friends, you need some friends at those levels. If we don't have connection at the deeper levels, we tend to try and focus on trying to create deep connection without the foundation that makes that connection safe. This often leads to intensity rather than true intimacy in connection and creates relationships that don't have strong foundations, so we get hurt more often.

Exercise 9–1:

1. Approximately how many people do you have at each of the four levels (close friends, good friends, general friendships, and meaningful connections)?
2. How much of what you know about yourself do you share with those you are closest to?
3. How does what you share with good friends differ from what you share with close friends?
4. Do you feel comfortable with how many people you have at each level? What would you like to change, if anything?

Relational Currency

A metaphor that can be helpful when setting boundaries around how and what you share with others is relational currency. I have fake money in a cabinet at my office that I use to help clients walk through visualizing this concept. Consider that what we share about ourselves, our lives, and our experiences can be viewed as having different vulnerability values. For example, anyone who has met me or even looked at my bio online knows I have six children. That piece of information might be a $1 item for me. I don't consider it private information at all. Talking about my relationship with my children would have a higher value. Discussing any struggles I've gone through as a mother would be an even higher value. Often, we can tell if a relationship feels balanced or imbalanced, but we have a hard time explaining why. Considering the relationship from the viewpoint of relational currency can help you to understand the balance in relationships better. It also allows for the relational balance to be based on different areas. We may not invest in a relationship in the same way as another person might, but the level of investment overall might be similar.

When considering how balanced relationships are, I'd start by asking yourself "how much am I putting down?" and "how much are they putting down?" Picture the relationship as a table and relational investments are like putting money down on the table. What level of information are you sharing and what type are they sharing? How much energy are you putting into the relationship and how much energy are they putting into the relationship?

Recognize that most relationships are built over time. The balance in the relationship isn't necessarily about what's being exchanged in any specific moment, but about the account balance throughout the history of the relationship. There will be times when we have more energy to give and other times when we're more drained or focused on something else. Long-term relationships are about balance over time.

This tool can also be used to build healthy relationships and understand what limits to set within them. If you've been hurt by others or if you've struggled with problematic patterns of escape behaviors, it can be scary to work toward connecting with others. If you grew up in a family with dysfunctional roles and rules, you may have been taught that you don't deserve to connect with others or that no one is interested in connecting with you. Hopefully the work you've done so far has helped you to see that you are a valuable person and worthy of connection. This tool can help you understand how to build connection with others in a structured way.

I use this as a group exercise. I hand out fake money that is blank on the back and have people write down information about themselves that might be at each level – $1 items, $5 items, $10 items, etc. This helps us understand how to share in a balanced way and build healthy connection with others.

When you're building a relationship, start with lower dollar amounts. When we share things about ourselves, it's the equivalent to sitting down at a table with someone and putting money on the table. If we put down $5, they might match it with $5 of their own, put down less, maybe a $1 item, put down more, like a $10 item, or they could take our $5 and get up and walk away. Starting by sharing $5 lowers our risk of being abandoned. As the relationship develops, gradually you can choose to share higher value items, and see what the other person does in response. If they match the value by sharing parts of themselves at the same level, or if they share something at a slightly higher level, then you can choose to move to that level of connection. If they don't match it, meaning if they share something at a lower level or don't offer anything, then I'd recommend stepping back what you're offering. If that happens repeatedly, then you may have reached the maximum connection you can currently build with them.

Relational currency can also be used to decide how to respond to someone. I often have clients come into sessions asking how to respond to emails or texts. I have them consider the dollar amount being offered. Then I have them decide if they want to match it, raise it, or lower it.

Exercise 9–2:

1. What might a $1, $5, or $10 piece of information about you include?
2. What would a $100, $500, or $1000 piece of information about you be?
3. Have you experienced relationships where you felt you were consistently giving more than you were getting back? Consider one of those relationships through the lens of relational currency. How does that impact the way you view the relationship?
4. What were you taught by your family about how much you should give and how much you should expect from others?

Call and Respond

We've talked about what to share and levels of relational connection. Let's discuss how to share. Have you ever heard the term "call and respond"? It's a musical term. You're likely familiar with it, even if you don't know the term. Have you ever seen a movie that includes a military group marching, where the leader sings a line, and the group echoes it back?

Usually something like "I don't know, but I've been told." The pattern of the leader saying something and the group echoing it back is "call and respond." The way this translates to healthy communication is called reflective listening.

The term "reflective listening" indicates the goal of reflecting back what we've heard without putting our thoughts or emotions into it. If you look into a mirror, you'll see yourself, not someone else. Emotionally focused therapy uses "enactments" to structure healthy and empathetic sharing (Johnson, 2004, 2008). Enactments are the structure EFT-trained therapists use to help their clients express their emotions and needs and hear the emotions and needs of others. Enactments involve taking turns reflectively listening.

Combining all of this together, the structure of healthy communication involves **taking turns** sharing each person's emotions, needs, and experiences, while the other person or persons involved in the conversation reflect back what they're hearing, without adding their opinions or thoughts, to ensure that they understand what the person sharing is saying. Once everything has been shared, then the same process can be used for solutions.

This starts with processing your emotions and needs so you can share them clearly and in a way that honors yourself and others. Use the tools we discussed in Chapter 6 to consider your emotions and the needs behind them. Stay in your hula hoop as we talked about in Chapter 8. Depending on the energy behind what you're feeling, it may be helpful to process your emotions and needs with someone else before having a conversation with the person or people your energy is connected to. It may be helpful to write your thoughts down.

Once you've done the foundational work to understand your "song" (referring to the call and respond metaphor), set up a time to talk. Be clear about what you're asking for, especially if it's a situation where those you're talking to might need time to process through their own emotions and needs. Before you start the conversation, set up the format, meaning explain that you'd like to take turns reflectively listening. Consider steps each of you can take throughout the process to redirect the conversation back to the call and respond format. For example, if someone has an emotional reaction to what someone else says and starts presenting their own thoughts on the topic before the other person is finished sharing, you might say "It's my turn now. Can you please reflect what you're hearing me say? I'd be happy to listen to you when I'm done."

As each of you take turns sharing, focus on staying in your hula hoop and sharing your emotions, needs, and experiences. Often phrases like "the message I received, whether or not you meant to send it, was..." can help us advocate for ourselves without telling someone else what they did or said. The more you can focus on your emotions, needs, and experience, and the less you focus on the specific details, the more effective the conversation will be. Talking about details usually leads to arguments about what happened instead of working through the experience, as you will likely not be able to process the experience together until each of you agrees about the specific details. In Chapter 3 we discussed Gordon's I-statements (1970). That's a good starting point for sharing. To remind you, I-statements sound something like "When ____ happened, the message I got was ____, which makes me feel____." That phrase can start the process of sharing, but I recommend going deeper with what you've experienced.

While one person shares, the other or others reflectively listen. The most basic form of reflective listening is repeating back what someone says but using different words to make sure you understand what they're talking about. Remember, you're not putting your emotions, needs, or thoughts into that part of the conversation. Try to incorporate empathy, which involves putting yourself into their shoes. We'll talk more about empathy in the next chapter.

Reflective listening isn't about agreeing with someone's perspective, it's about hearing them. Remember that emotions are valid. Don't try to logically argue someone out of what they are feeling. Don't be defensive. This isn't about being right, it's about understanding each other. The better you understand each other, the more quickly you'll resolve the conflict and the more effective your solution will be. In my experience, listening, really listening, to each other resolves about 80% of any conflict. It's like putting all of each person's cards on the table – if you can see every card, you have the best chance of coming up with a solution that matches them all. Also, if each person is given time and space to share what they're feeling, they don't have to keep fighting to be heard.

As each person shares, reflect back what is heard. Pause them to reflect if it feels like you've hit your limit with what you can remember and reflect. This is sort of like going to a buffet. You can only fit so much on your plate. You need to empty what's on the plate before getting more or the food falls off. As you reflect, ask "is that right?" and give them space to consider and respond. Often the answer to this question will be "no, not exactly." Sometimes this is because the information wasn't understood and sometimes it will be because once it's reflected, the person sharing might realize that the information isn't exactly what they meant. Again, the goal is to understand each other. This isn't about criticizing or having to phrase things perfectly the first time. After reflecting, ask "is there anything else?"

Once one person is done, switch roles to give someone else a chance to share. Make sure each person has time and space to share what they are feeling and thinking. Often this process requires multiple turns for each person. Keep talking until each of you feels heard and understood, then work on the solution if one has not become apparent.

Use the same steps as you consider the solution. Take turns sharing potential solutions and use reflective listening to ensure you understand what others are suggesting. Often potential solutions will incorporate some pieces of the puzzle but need tweaks to address the situation completely. Honor the work each person puts into the solution, rather than criticizing them, as you talk through any changes needed.

Exercise 9–3:

1. Think of a recent time you had a disagreement with someone or experienced pain as a result of interpersonal connection. Write down your feelings and thoughts about it. Use I-statements, focus on your emotions and general needs rather than solutions, stay in your hula hoop, and consider the messages you got. Include the least amount of details possible; focus on explaining your experience instead of arguing about what happened.
2. Consider what you wrote for question 1. How was this different from the way you usually present information? Did it feel any different? Did it sound different?
3. What have you learned about yourself from the last two questions?
4. What steps can you take to incorporate these tools into your conversations?

Super Short Summary:

Sharing with others in a healthy way helps to build relationships and keeps us emotionally safe. Understanding the different levels of connection we have helps us to know how much to share. It's helpful to be aware of how much we're investing in each relationship and how much we're getting back, as well as what level we're sharing at. Balanced and healthy communication includes processing through what we feel and think as well as listening to what others feel and think.

Chapter Questions:

1. What did you connect to the most in this chapter?
2. What steps are you taking to apply this material to your life?

Chapter 10

Connection
Developing and Expressing Empathy

Adding the fifth component of the Connected Recovery® model, connection in middle recovery relates to using the tools we've worked on to develop and express empathy. The word "empathy" comes from the German word "Einfühlung," which means "feeling into." A German psychologist named Theodor Lipps used it in 1903 to describe the process of projecting oneself into someone else's experience. Edward Titchener translated the word into English in 1909 and explained it as the way we understand and resonate with someone else's emotions by trying to see an experience through their eyes. As we talked about in Chapter 3, empathy is understanding someone else's pain by connecting it to emotions you've experienced.

One reason we wait until this point in the process to dive into empathy is that empathy requires that we understand our own emotions and process through the experiences we've had. If you were taught that you weren't allowed to feel, or that your emotions didn't matter, it was likely difficult for you to really feel your emotions. This might have happened in your family-of-origin, or it might have happened in relationships you were part of as an adult, or both. If you developed a pattern of escape behaviors in order to deal with the pain you'd gone through, you numbed your emotions, possibly for years or even decades, which makes it very difficult to understand them.

The foundation for empathy comes from understanding our own emotions and experiences. As we talked about in Chapter 6, emotions aren't bad or good. They provide us with information. Empathy takes emotions a step further, using emotions to help develop and strengthen connection to ourselves and others.

Empathy is sitting with someone in their pain. It's not trying to tell them they shouldn't be in pain. It's not sitting outside and being glad it's not you. It's not judging them for being in pain. It's not telling them how to stop feeling pain or telling them what worked for you. It's sitting with them.

Shortly after my last baby was born, I was diagnosed with heart failure. I was 34. As I went through treatment for my condition, it was interesting to watch how people responded to knowing what I was going through. Some people avoided me. They didn't know what to do and it felt like they didn't want to acknowledge that something like that could happen, potentially because they didn't want to be afraid it would happen to them. It was painful to see people notice me and deliberately avoid me, but I could understand that. I didn't want it to be real, but I didn't have the option of opting out of dealing with it.

DOI: 10.4324/9781003623359-13

Others seem to feed on the drama and look at it as juicy gossip. Some pitied me. Both of those responses were very difficult for me to deal with. The responses that were most help-ful were the empathetic responses, people who said "I don't even know what to say. You matter. Let me know if I can help." I remember one person, who I didn't know very well, hearing about some particularly bad news I'd received and coming up to me and saying "I heard. There is nothing else to say but 'this sucks.'" Empathy isn't having answers or trying to make someone feel better. It's sitting with them in the pain so they aren't alone.

Exercise 10–1:

1. Think of a time when you felt empathy for someone else. It can be related to a major situation or a minor one. What did that feel like?
2. Have you felt empathy from others? What did that feel like? How can you tell it's empathy?
3. What type of response do you have to seeing pain in others? Why do you think you have that response?

Empathy for Self

As we mentioned above, empathy starts with understanding your own emotions and pain. Many of the questions throughout this book have involved considering yourself and your experiences. As you've gone through those questions, have you started to see yourself and your experiences differently?

We often work to have empathy for others but believe it shouldn't apply to us. This might come from believing we aren't worthy of it (shame, which we talked about earlier), or believing what we've gone through isn't as bad as what others go through. When talk-ing about painful experiences, the vast majority of those I've talked to, both clients and connections outside of my office, make comments along the lines of "I know it's not as bad as what others go through" or "it could've been worse." There will almost always be a way a situation could have been worse. That doesn't change that the situation hurt you. Sometimes it can be helpful to recognize that a situation could have been worse, but don't start with that, and don't end with it as that minimizes your pain and prevents you from processing it.

Emotional Awareness

There are four steps that might be helpful in feeling empathy for yourself. The first step is emotional awareness. In the previous chapter, we talked about hearing other people with-out judgment. How often do you stop and listen to yourself and let yourself finish process-ing something before you just try to find a solution or shut the emotion down?

Find a method that lets you feel your pain. Journaling or writing letters (don't send them without doing additional work to decide if you really want to share them) often helps. Sometimes art can help as well. Music has a lot of emotions connected to it. I have playlists on my phone that express different emotions, for example one for when I'm feeling drained, one for when I'm mad, one for when I'm excited about something, one for when I need to have confidence. One of my clients created a "f you" playlist filled with songs that helped them process through the pain they were feeling regarding a specific situation. They shared it with other group members and others in the group created their own playlists. Some used heavier music and others used music that expressed the same emotions in a soft-sounding way. Find something that helps you feel your emotions in the way that's right for you.

Perspective-Taking

If it's difficult for you to consider your pain, it might be helpful to first consider what you might feel about someone else going through the experience. This is one of the benefits of group therapy. When clients who are group members downplay the pain of their experiences, often they'll be more able to see the pain if I ask them what they would think if someone else in group had gone through whatever they are processing.

Also, make sure you're taking age into account. Consider what you would feel if the situation were to happen to anyone else the age you were when you experienced the situation. Don't judge your past self by your current knowledge and abilities. Using this approach can help minimize shame, which can send us the message that we aren't worthy of empathy. Your emotions are valid!

They also likely make sense in context. Emotions happen for a reason. They give us information about what's going on and how it's impacting us and others. You aren't crazy for feeling what you feel and there's a reason you feel that way. Recognizing your emotions as valid helps you to receive the information they provide.

Non-Judgmental Acceptance

When considering why we had the emotional response we had, we realize that we may have reacted to a miscommunication or a mistranslation of a situation. In some cases, we also might recognize that our response to our reaction doesn't align with who we want to be. Guess what? You're human. You're going to make mistakes. You don't have to be perfect for your emotions to be valid.

If you react to a misconception, give yourself time and space to process the emotion you felt. Merely telling yourself that your response was based on inaccurate information won't erase the impact what you thought happened had on you. If your response to an emotion doesn't align with who you want to be, take steps to make amends to yourself and anyone else impacted by it, but don't ignore the emotions underneath your response. Recognizing that you made a mistake in the way you respond doesn't change your emotions.

Self-Compassion

Treat yourself kindly. In her book about self-compassion, Kristin Neff (2011) highlights the importance of being gentle and understanding with ourselves. She highlights that self-blame and judgment are not helpful and that pain and imperfection are universal human experiences. You aren't alone. She also states that being present with your emotions, rather than repressing or exaggerating them, allows you to process them in a balanced way.

This step brings the other three steps together into action. As we allow ourselves to acknowledge our emotions, consider what the experience might be like for someone else, and stop judging ourselves for being human, we can make space to care for ourselves. I call this step "mothering" yourself. I recognize that you may not have not had healthy experiences with your mother. When I use the term "mothering," I'm referring to how you should have been treated. How a mother would treat their child if the mother had done the work to minimize their dysfunction and provide a supportive environment for their child. Consider what you need in the situation. Do you need rest, do you need support? What would make your day easier? Consider the list of bucket-fillers you made when reading through the introduction. What scents might help make your day better, what tastes might help, what sounds might feel comforting, what could you incorporate physically or visually to make yourself feel cared for?

Exercise 10–2:

1. What response do you usually have toward yourself when you feel pain?
2. Who taught you to respond that way?
3. What does self-compassion look like for you in daily life? What small, tangible acts help you feel cared for?

Empathy for Others

True empathy for self creates a foundation that helps us to heal and increases our ability to connect with others. The relationship we've cultivated with ourselves extends outward toward others in our lives and the communities we're part of. Empathy for self helps to reduce shame, self-criticism, and insecurity. When we believe that we matter, we also can better understand that others matter as well, and we can work to find a balance that helps us advocate for ourselves and connect with others. The work we do to develop emotional attunement and non-judgmental acceptance for ourselves often naturally integrates into our interpersonal interactions.

According to Daniel Goleman (1995), a psychologist who popularized the concept of emotional intelligence, there are three elements to empathy for others: cognitive empathy, affective empathy, and compassionate empathy. Cognitive empathy is the ability to understand someone else logically. Affective empathy is the capacity to feel someone else's emotions. Compassionate empathy uses both logical and emotional connection to take action to connect to someone else.

Empathy for others is not just about understanding someone else's feelings, but also about using that understanding to connect with them. It helps us to stay grounded as we work through conflict with others as we can more easily see where they are coming from and understand how the situation might have impacted them. As we discussed in the previous chapter when we talked about reflective listening, understanding where someone is coming from does not necessarily mean we agree with them or that we think their reactions were appropriate responses. It means we can better understand what the experience was like for them. This can help us to depersonalize their behaviors, decreasing the impact those behaviors have on us.

Empathy doesn't weaken or eliminate boundaries. It helps us better understand how to maintain boundaries, especially when we combine empathy for self with empathy for others. Empathy helps us to recognize underlying needs of each person, including ourselves, allowing us to address those needs more effectively. It helps us to recognize that each person's feelings and experiences matter.

Empathy is not always easy, even when you've done the work to develop the skills and emotional muscles needed to practice it. Recognize that while empathy deepens connections and adds to your life, it can also drain you emotionally. This is not always the case as sometimes the connection that comes from expressing empathy fills your emotional bucket more than the efforts to have empathy drained it. Be aware of the potential cost of empathy though and consider steps you might need to replenish your bucket after empathetic connection.

Exercise 10–3:

1. Is cognitive empathy (logical understanding) or affective empathy (emotional connection) easier for you? Why?
2. How do you differentiate between empathizing with someone and taking responsibility for their emotions?
3. How can you create a balance between being empathetic and protecting your emotional well-being?

Steps to Expressing Empathy

Expressing empathy is sitting with someone in their pain. There are three questions you can ask yourself when working to understand the pain someone else is sitting in. The first question is "what might they be feeling?" You can use the emotions chart for this if needed. If they want to talk, you can also ask them. Empathy focuses on meeting them where they are at, not forcing them to open up. A good way to ask is "Is there anything you'd like to share about what's going on?"

As you consider what they might be feeling, ask yourself if you've ever felt something similar. Focus on other times you've felt the same emotions as well as other times you've gone through similar situations. Realize that your experience might not be exactly the same, but it can help give you context. Make sure that you don't make the situation about you though. Don't say "I know exactly how you feel" because you don't, even if you've gone through something very similar. Instead use language that creates space for them to have their own experience, such as "I can imagine how you might feel."

Additionally, recognize that there are two different elements that help shape how a person experiences something. In his discussion around empathetic understanding, Carl Rogers (1957), a psychologist who developed the Person-Centered Therapy model, highlighted the importance of considering both generalized empathy and person-specific empathy. Generalized empathy refers to the universal aspects of the human experience, or what it might be like for anyone to go through the situation. Person-specific empathy considers how a person's individual history and their specific, unique personal experiences impact the situation.

Finally, consider what the situation might feel like if it were you. Think about the potential influence of external factors as well as the primary issue. How might other current issues in their life amplify or alter their experience? Imagine what emotions you might have and what support and resources would help you feel understood and supported.

The above work can help you shift into a space where you can provide empathetic support, although you can't know exactly what they might want in the moment. I recommend asking something like "Do you want to talk through it? Or just have me listen? Or do you want someone to just be there with you? Is there something I can do for you or get for you that would help?" Don't try to fix it by coming up with solutions for them. Don't minimize it by saying something that starts with "at least..." or saying "it's not that bad." Don't make it about you. If you've gone through something similar and you think it might help them to know that, say as little as possible about your experience to convey what you went through. This is about them.

While this may seem complicated, putting it into action is often very simple. It can be as simple as:

"How are you doing?"
"Today was rough."
"Do you want to talk about it?"
"No, thanks."
"Ok. Can I just sit with you?"
"Why?"
"Because I've had difficult days and sometimes it just helps to know you're not alone."

In this interaction, the first person asked what their friend wanted, listened to their response, considered when they had gone through something similar, offered a very brief statement explaining the connection they made to what their friend was going through, and let the friend know they were seen and loved. That's the goal of empathy – for the person it's focused on to feel seen, heard, and valued.

Exercise 10–4:

1. When have you expressed empathy for someone? How did that experience impact your connection with them?
2. Think of a time when you or someone you loved experienced something painful. How might you view that situation through generalized empathy, meaning what anyone going through it might feel?
3. Using the same example, how might you view the situation through person-specific empathy, meaning why it might have been painful for them specifically because of what they've experienced?
4. How does the example conversation reflect the core principles of empathy?

Wrapping Up Middle Recovery

The steps of middle recovery help to create deeper emotional understanding around yourself, where you came from, and how you relate to others. They also help you balance connection between yourself and others. By learning to identify and process your emotions, you better understand the needs behind them. This helps to decrease pain as you are better able to resolve them. It helps you to move beyond basic safety into deeper authentic connection.

True connection is not at the expense of yourself or at the expense of those connected to you. The work we've done in this phase includes self-advocacy as well as empathy for self and others. The tools in this section help strengthen boundaries and create healthier relational dynamics. The tools help you to develop a clearer understanding of yourself and work toward connection that is grounded, intentional, and mutually respectful.

As you work to better understand the insights you developed about yourself and implement the relational tools you've been introduced to, remember that this is about progress, not perfection. It's a continuous journey. Practice empathy for yourself as you continue to learn and grow. It will be challenging but also rewarding. By honoring your emotions, recognizing your needs, and approaching yourself and your connection to others with empathy and authenticity, you can create meaningful and lasting change that benefits both you and those you care about.

Super Short Summary:

Empathy is understanding what someone (including yourself) is feeling and sitting with them in their pain. It's important to have empathy for yourself as well as empathy for others. Empathy can be divided into two categories: generalized empathy, which means what anyone would feel in that situation, and person-specific empathy, which refers to how a person's experiences might make a situation particularly painful for them.

Chapter Questions:

1. What did you connect to the most in this chapter?
2. What steps are you taking to apply this material to your life?

Restore – Healing Sexuality

Education

Defining Healthy Sexuality

The final phase of recovery is healing sexuality. This refers to understanding yourself and your experiences at the deepest level. It is not about having more sex or incorporating different aspects into your sex life. It's about getting to know who you are at your core, learning to be confident, and learning to love yourself. The education component of late recovery is about defining healthy sexuality.

Don't feel that you need to be ready to take the steps outlined in this section of the book just because you've read the previous chapters. It's ok if you are reading this phase just to get the information and aren't ready to apply the tools we talk about. In general, I find that recovery (becoming whole) happens in layers. It's ok to take what connects to you now and come back to it later to deepen the work you do in this area. Actually, it's not just ok, it's really important to address it at the level you are at now. Don't push yourself to do something you don't feel safe with or ready for.

Considering sexuality from the perspective of the Hierarchy of Needs we discussed in Chapter 6, healthy sexuality is a more advanced need. This means that the lower sections of the hierarchy need to be fairly solid. We need to have the basics for survival of course, such as air, water, food, and shelter. We need to have safety in our lives. Not only physical safety, but also emotional safety, basic financial security, and stability, along with justice and trust. If we don't feel safe, it is very difficult to have the capacity to feel confidence and joy. We need to feel supported as well. We need connection with self and others, a feeling of belonging combined with friendship and family, whatever our "family" looks like, meaning it can be a family we build rather than those we are related to by birth or marriage. We need empathy for self and others, and we need to have connections we can be vulnerable with. We need to have an understanding of our inherent self-worth, along with the confidence to believe our experiences and embrace our emotions and needs.

Exercise 11–1:

1. What fears or concerns do you have about navigating this phase of recovery?
2. What level do you feel comfortable setting for yourself as you go through this section? What support or boundaries do you need to make it safe for you to consider information related to sexuality?
3. How might you know if you need to pause reading through this and come back to it later? What steps do you need to take if you hit that point?

DOI: 10.4324/9781003623359-15

Personalizing Your Definition

When I first started developing my material around healthy sexuality, I mentioned it to another therapist. I told her I was trying to figure out what healthy sexuality was. She said something along the lines of "you know, feeling sexy isn't about sex." At the time, her statement didn't quite make sense to me. I knew she was right but couldn't quite understand why or what it meant.

I thought about her comment for several weeks. One evening a couple of my sessions cancelled. I was working from home that night and my kids were over at my sister's house. I went out and asked my husband on a date. This was in the middle of Covid, so a date meant getting take-out. When we were in the parking lot, we realized that our car had a burned-out headlight. My husband popped the hood and tried to remove the bulb so we could replace it with the spare we kept in the car, but he couldn't figure out how to get the bulb out.

Between the two of us, I'm the one with the engineer's mind. I pulled up a YouTube video on my phone, watched the first 15 seconds of it, hopped out of the car, and removed the burned-out bulb. I was dressed in my work clothes, which included slacks, a sweater, and heels, and it was cold, so I had my leather jacket on. Standing in the parking lot, having just figured out how to fix something I had previously known nothing about, in clothes I felt confident in, I realized I felt sexy. It had nothing to do with anyone else watching me. It had nothing to do with sex. It had to do with being me. Years ago, I heard a presenter who was a sex therapist at a conference. I don't remember who she was, but I remember her saying something about people feeling sexy when they did things they loved and did them well. This experience aligned with that.

The aspects of my experiences won't be the same as yours as you figure out what healthy sexuality is for you. Everyone is different. It will have the same level of connection to self though. In her 2016 TED Talk, Emily Nagoski, a sex educator, says that the keys to a happy sex life are confidence and joy. "Confidence is knowing what's true. Joy is loving what's true."

Healthy sexuality is about a deep connection with yourself. It's not about the physical act of sex, although that can certainly be part of what you do with your sexuality. It's about knowing who you are. Knowing what you like and don't like. Knowing your strengths and weaknesses. Knowing your quirks and struggles. Knowing who you are and learning not just to accept, but to love that person. Healthy sexuality is the deepest level of connection to yourself and your body. It includes the ability to share that connection, when sharing is relationally safe, in ways that allow you and those you choose to connect with to be fully present. It looks different for every person and every relationship.

At the very beginning of this journey, in the introduction, we defined healthy sexual behaviors. Just like the definition of healthy sexuality, healthy sexual behaviors will be different for each individual and each relationship. As stated in the introduction, healthy sexual behaviors are behaviors that align with your moral values, allow you to fulfill the commitments you've made to yourself or others, encourage growth, development, and well-being for you and others, ensure the safety and well-being of yourself and others, show respect to yourself and others, and strengthen congruency and authenticity.

Exercise 11–2:

1. When do you feel most confident about yourself? What influences that? For example, are there specific styles of clothing, specific activities?
2. What do you love about yourself? What do you struggle to love about yourself?

Shame and Sexuality

Another important aspect of healthy sexuality is addressing shame. By this, I don't just mean shame as we've talked about it throughout this book, although that is an important part of the equation. To love ourselves and who we are, we need to believe we are worthy of love and belonging, using Brené Brown's language related to shame (2012). In relation to sexuality, we need to address shame in regard to sexuality in general.

Many authors discuss shame as it relates to sex. Siegel (2019) highlights that even treatments related to problematic sexual behaviors avoid discussing sex and only focus on the unhealthy patterns. Outside of basic human sexuality classes, I'm not aware of any therapy or counseling schools that incorporate education around sex, even programs that focus specifically on treating relationships. Sex therapy is viewed as a completely different field of study.

As a society in general, we view sex as dirty. We separate it from other aspects of life and either don't talk about it, joke about it, or discuss it in a scholarly manner. We hide tampons or condoms beneath other items in our shopping carts. We don't talk to our kids about it and don't have real conversations about it with our friends. Fetishes, kink, and BDSM (sexual interactions involving power exchange) are viewed as deviant behaviors. Many religions teach "abstinence before marriage," but they often don't teach abstinence through education, they teach it through shame. I've heard of lessons that used chewed gum, white flowers dipped in black ink, large stains on white dresses, and nails hammered into boards as examples of how having sex before marriage impacts your value. When we do talk about it, it is usually one of two extremes. One is with disgust. The other is bragging about conquests. Sexual trauma is dismissed, minimized, or those who have been abused or attacked are blamed.

Sexual content is now widely available to anyone with an electronic device, but we don't talk to our kids about it and rarely talk about it in a balanced way with our trusted friends and significant others. We aren't given space to process or learn about sex or romance in a healthy way. For many, sex ed comes from mainstream porn. I have no idea where the original quote came from, but "learning about sex from mainstream porn is like learning to drive from Grand Theft Auto." The situations are extreme, consent is not taught, nor are normal elements of human sexual interaction. Romance novels focus on extremes as well. Even media that isn't porn or romance focuses on idealized interactions at inhuman levels. Hallmark Christmas movies and Disney movies end with happily ever after and we're taught to look for soulmates, people who will meet all of our needs. One of my friends talked to me about dating when the Twilight (Meyer, 2005) series came out. He said it was difficult to date because girls his age were looking for someone like Edward, who had the emotional intelligence of someone over 100 years old, the body of a boy in his late teens, who had to fight against his most basic instincts and needs every second to be with the girl he loved.

This isn't said to criticize any of the media I mentioned above. Temporarily escaping into worlds where we can have everything we want and we don't have to factor in real-life issues can be fun. The issue is when we don't see it as fake. We've talked about shame going between extremes; you have to be perfect, or you suck as a human being. Because we don't talk about sex or sexuality in a balanced way, we often have a shame-based view of sex and romance. Everything has to be perfect (not humanly possible) or it's wrong, we're wrong, and our relationships are wrong. We aren't given space to understand ourselves and determine what we like, who we are sexually and romantically, and honor the way our experiences have impacted those definitions.

Exercise 11–3:

1. Do you feel shame in relation to sex? Why or why not?
2. What was your education around sex like? Where did you learn about sex? What did you learn?

Accelerator and Brakes

The Dual Control Model was created in the 1990s at the Kinsey Institute by John Bancroft and Eric Jansen (1999). Emily Nagoski explains it in detail in her book, *Come As You Are* (2021), which focuses on understanding female sexuality (although a lot of the material applies to everyone), and her TED Talk (2016), and made it accessible and easily understood by using the terms "Accelerator" and "Brakes." She just published a book for relationships in 2024 called *Come Together*. I highly recommend reading her books and listening to her TED talks for more detailed information on this topic and on other topics related to healthy sexuality.

A basic understanding of the concept is vital for healthy sexual connection. If you were to try to drive a car and both the accelerator and brakes were being pushed at the same time, you wouldn't get very far. I don't have a whole lot of knowledge around car mechanics, but I think you'd probably burn the engine out at some point. If you want the car to actually go somewhere, you need to figure out how to balance between using the brake and using the accelerator. It would be next to impossible to get anywhere safely without using each when needed. That concept is also true for sexuality.

Getting to know yourself and believe the information your emotions are sending you involves not only understanding what you want and like, but also what you dislike, don't want, and don't feel comfortable with. Considering both aspects without judgment is critical, although you probably won't be able to do that, at least initially. In Phase 1, we looked at trauma responses and escape patterns and learned to see those with empathy for ourselves. In Phase 2, we considered emotions and needs, along with family-of-origin dynamics. Now, in Phase 3, we're addressing a potential additional layer of shame and pain, what we feel in connection to sexuality.

For those who have struggled with patterns of problematic sexual behavior, shame and fear connected to their behaviors often feel intrinsically linked to sexuality. Those who have been betrayed frequently have shame and fear related to sexuality. Additionally, anyone who has gone through sexual abuse at any point in their life likely struggles with shame and fear at some level around sexuality as well.

Fear and shame are powerful. And it makes sense if you feel them. One of my favorite quotes by Emily Nagoski (yes, I quote her a lot, she's awesome) is "whatever you're experiencing in your sexuality… is the result of your sexual response mechanism functioning appropriately… in an inappropriate world" (2021, p. 9). You've survived what you've been through. You weren't destroyed. Of course you were impacted by it. Your sexuality is still there, possibly covered by mounds of shame and/or fear. You aren't so broken that you will never be whole again.

Healing is not about forcing yourself to ignore everything you've gone through that leads you to push on your "brakes." One of the most significant issues that push on the "brakes" is shame over their lack of connection to sexuality, over the shame and fear they feel in this arena. The first step toward connecting to yourself is to recognize and accept your current level of connection and safety (or lack of connection and safety) in this area. Don't try to push yourself to ignore those emotions and the boundaries you've set up for yourself internally and possibly interpersonally.

Exercise 11–4:

1. What is your current level of connection and safety in relation to exploring your sexuality?
2. How do you feel about where you're at in this process?

Key Dimensions of Healthy Sexuality

According to the World Health Organization (n.d.), sexual health includes four domains: physical, emotional, mental, and social. Each of these is important to consider.

Physical

If you are dealing with physical issues related to sexuality, consult a physician. One physical issue related to sexuality might include unwanted pain during sex. Very often there are steps that can address pain related to sexual interactions, but many people are embarrassed to talk about it. If you like golfing and your arm or shoulder hurts when you golf, you'd probably talk to a doctor about it. If you run regularly and your feet or legs hurt during or afterwards, you'd probably talk to a doctor about it. Due to widespread societal shame around sex, it can feel more taboo to talk about physical pain related to sex.

A sex therapist may also be able to help. They can help you consider different positions or steps related to sexual connection that might minimize or eliminate any pain. Other physical conditions can impact pain during sex. For example, medical conditions related to the lower back or hips can make some sexual positions more painful. Additionally, a better understanding of physical arousal and foreplay often helps. Tools such as lubricant can help as well. If you look for a lubricant, look for one that is either silicone-based or water-based.

Be aware that sometime pain related to sex can be connected to emotional and mental impacts. Our bodies can convey messages to us that we may try and mentally push past. At the same time, recognize that our bodies may respond in ways that don't align with what we want or desire. This is called "arousal non-concordance." We'll talk about that in more detail in the next chapter.

Don't push your body to do something that's hurting you in a way you don't want to be hurt. Talk to a physician or a sex therapist or both to better understand if the pain is physical or emotional or both. As we've discussed the earlier steps in recovery, one aspect we've highlighted over and over is believing yourself and the messages your heart and mind are sending. Believe the messages your body is sending as well and listen to them. Spend the time to sort through your physical responses to find answers that fit best for you.

Emotional and Mental

The emotional and mental domains often overlap. Emotions and logic work together to give us the most complete set of information for our decisions and responses (Levine, 2022). As we talked about earlier, emotions send us information. Often, we consider emotions less accurate, but the information we get from our emotions is just as valid and valuable as logical conclusions. Both instinct and logic help us to create safety in our environment and build connection with ourselves and others.

Emotions help us understand what we feel about something. Logic can help us explain why we feel that way. Both can take work to explore. The tools we discussed throughout this book, specifically in Chapter 6, can help deepen our understanding of our emotions. The steps we've walked through to make sense of our experiences can help us make sense of the emotions we experience. The most accurate information and deepest understanding of ourselves and our connection to others comes from a combination of both. Just as with physical responses, believe your emotions. Pay attention to the logic connected to those. Everything makes sense in context. Don't dismiss yourself or what you feel or think. Tying this back to accelerators and brakes, listening to your emotions and understanding your thoughts helps you to decide when to push on or release the pressure you're putting on the brakes or the accelerator. Both help you to determine boundaries you need or steps you want to take.

Social

The social domain of sexuality includes how your understanding of your sexual self, behaviors connected to that part of you, and your relationships are influenced by societal, cultural, and interpersonal factors. What have you been taught you are supposed to be or act like? What have you learned about what relationships look like? What have you been taught you were supposed to like/enjoy or not like/enjoy? It also includes what you learned about sexuality and sexual health, including consent and safety. It impacts how you communicate your needs and boundaries and how you perceive power dynamics in relationships, along with what you're allowed to talk about and how you're allowed to talk about it. The social aspect of sexuality incorporates any biases or stigma. Often it is highly influenced by media, which can educate and/or misinform. Finally, it includes sexual rights and access to physical resources.

What we've been taught and what we've learned can either support healthy sexual expression or create shame and confusion around it. Sometimes we get different information from different parts of our lives. Our parents might teach us something different than what we learn from friends or the media. Perhaps relationships you had taught you something different than what you learned growing up. All of our experiences shape us. Keep in mind that messages can be overt or covert. You absolutely can learn to say or not say things, do or not do things, based on covert messaging.

Connection Between All Four

Each of these facets of sexual health are intertwined. Social messages can impact emotion, specifically in relation to shame or confidence. Those messages often are foundational in our belief about our right to have emotions or thoughts or take action in regard to our sexuality. Our emotions and social messages can prevent us from being able to reach out about issues related to the physical aspect of sexual health. Societal influences and the protection of our sexual rights often have a significant impact on our emotional and physical sexual health.

Exercise 11–5:

1. Consider the physical aspects of your sexual health – what concerns or struggles have you had, or do you currently have, in this area?
2. How do you think emotions and logic impact your connection to your sexual self?
3. How have social influences impacted you in regard to sexuality?

Super Short Summary:

Healthy sexuality isn't about having more sex. It's about connecting to yourself on a deep level and loving who you are. Each person's definition of what is sexy for them will be different. Often shame is connected to sexuality. Understanding that shame can help us process through it. It's important to understand what you like and what you don't like because both are part of who you are. Sexuality includes physical, emotional, mental, and social domains.

Chapter Questions:

1. What did you connect to the most in this chapter?
2. What steps are you taking to apply this material to your life?

Honesty

Identifying and Processing Sexual Trauma

The last chapter began our discussion around how what we've gone through has impacted our connection to our sexual selves. We talked about trauma in general in Chapters 1 and 2, and relational and family-of-origin patterns in Chapter 7. The honesty component of late recovery focuses on identifying and processing sexual trauma. As with every step of this process, we're deepening the work you've already done, using similar tools. Due to the stigma and shame connected to sexuality, along with the depth of emotional pain, we save processing sexual trauma for the last phase of recovery. **This topic can be particularly hard to handle.** Consider what type of support you need as you explore this topic. Be aware of the emotions that come up for you. Reach out for support to process through them. Don't push yourself to read through this if the emotions are too much to handle. Take it slow and give yourself time and space to process the information and connections you make. Recognize that whether or not you have personal experience with sexual abuse, it can be difficult to read about the topic.

Sometimes we don't realize that we have experienced sexual trauma or abuse. Just as we talked about in earlier chapters, new information can give us new insights into the experiences we've had. You may also realize that your behavior has been abusive toward someone else. Healing includes processing through what happened to us along with processing through what we've done to others. If your patterns have included abusive behaviors toward someone else, work to understand the truth of the situation, process through what led you to develop those patterns, process through your emotions, take the steps to make amends to those you have hurt and to change your behaviors going forward.

If you connect with this material, whether or not you know going into it that it applies directly to you, you will likely go through the stages of grief as you process it. As a reminder, grief often starts with shock. We cycle through anger, raw emotions, bargaining (how could I change the story so it has a different ending or different impact), making meaning, and acceptance. Acceptance isn't "I'm ok with this," it's "this is what it is, and this is how I'm moving forward." We don't experience those stages in order. At the beginning, there's a whole lot of shock and very little acceptance. At the end, there's a whole lot of acceptance and very little shock. The rest of it is a mix of everything. Even after processing through grief, we may still have flashes of the different stages. New realizations are often like having a new experience. Realizations at deeper levels may feel like new

DOI: 10.4324/9781003623359-16

experiences as well. Give yourself time and space to process through any realizations you have. Practice empathy for yourself. Get the support you need.

Exercise 12–1:

1. What concerns do you have about reading through this chapter?
2. How might you know if you need to reach out for support?
3. What steps can you take to get support if needed?

Sexual Abuse

The word "abuse" is fairly common, but it's one of those words that often we have a difficult time defining. Merriam-Webster's definition of abuse highlights that it includes wrong or excessive use, is an attack, is unjust, and is maltreatment (n.d.-a). Abuse causes harm or distress and often includes a power imbalance, meaning the person abusing someone else exerts control, manipulation, or coercion over the person being abused, violating their boundaries, autonomy, and well-being.

Sexual abuse refers to any non-consensual act or behavior imposed on an individual, regardless of the relationship between the individuals involved. Sexual abuse can occur across different contexts, including between adults, within families, in relationships, and among children.

Sexual abuse includes, but is not limited to the following:

- Unwanted sexual contact – Touching you or making you touch yourself or someone else without your consent.

  Note: Children cannot legally give consent to adults or individuals significantly older than they are (3+ years). Power dynamics can also reduce or eliminate a person's ability to consent, even in adult relationships.

- Non-contact sexual abuse – Making you watch or listen to sexual acts.
- Forced exposure to sexual content – Making you listen to, read, or view sexual material aimed at you or others.

  Note: Exposing children to sexually explicit material is a form of abuse.

- Indecent exposure – Exposing oneself or forcing someone else to expose sexual parts of themselves without consent.
- Violations of privacy – Watching, recording, photographing, or filming you without your knowledge and/or permission.
- Sharing intimate images without consent – Distributing sexual photos, audio, or videos of you as a minor, or without your knowledge and/or permission, whether as a minor or as an adult.

Note: Not all child sexual abuse comes from adults or even older children – children can abuse other children, particularly when there is a power imbalance, coercion, or lack of consent.

Sexual abuse can also occur within committed relationships, including marriages and long-term partnerships. Consent is essential in all relationships, and being in a relationship does not grant someone automatic access to another's body. Any of the above listed acts are abusive, even if they happen within relationships. There are some additional considerations within relationships. Below is a list of what sexual abuse in a relationship can include:

• Coercion and manipulation – Pressuring, guilt-tripping, or manipulating someone into sexual activity.
• Threats and intimidation – Using verbal threats or intimidation to force participation in sexual acts.
• Ignoring or violating boundaries – Refusing to respect a partner's physical or sexual boundaries.
• Non-consensual touching – Groping or touching without permission.
• Forcing sexual interactions – Up to and including rape.
• Secretly violating consent – Filming sexual encounters without permission or taking/sharing sexual photos without consent.

Sexual abuse can be deeply damaging, particularly when it occurs in relationships where safety and trust are expected. When I was growing up, we were taught about "stranger danger." Most sexual abuse doesn't come from strangers. Less than 20% of rapes are committed by a stranger and 93% of children and teen victims of sexual abuse knew the person who abused them (RAINN, n.d.). Knowing the person who sexually abused you often intensifies the emotional impact of the experience. Not only do you have to process emotions related to the abuse, but it's a breach of trust, a betrayal.

When abuse is committed by someone you know and trust, the emotional implications are often more complicated and confusing. Frequently there is a positive relational history, which can be difficult to reconcile with the abuse. This can cause mixed emotions, including anger, grief, guilt, or even love toward the person who abused you. The loss of emotional connection adds an additional layer to the pain. It can make it difficult to trust again, complicating recovery due to the struggle to let someone else in enough to get needed support.

Potential backlash can cause additional complications. Friends, family members, or even those in your community might pressure you to stay silent or blame you for what happened. This can be particularly true if the person who abused you holds a position of power and respect. Others connected to you may not believe you and may even retaliate against you for saying it happened. If you're abused by someone you know, setting boundaries for yourself about future interactions with them can be challenging. Even if the abuse is addressed, you may run into the person who abused you at future social events. This can make it difficult to create safety for yourself and can make it even more difficult to process through the abuse.

One topic that is often connected to identifying and processing through abuse is arousal. There are two distinct elements related to arousal. One is the way our bodies respond physically. The other is what we desire – what we want emotionally, mentally, and physically. Those don't always align.

Our bodies are wired to physically respond to sexual stimuli. If sexual parts of our bodies are touched, if we see or hear sexual material, or if we think of sexual situations, our bodies often respond physically. That doesn't always line up with what we want our bodies to do. This is called arousal non-concordance. Sometimes we want to be sexual, and our bodies don't respond the way we'd like them to. Those with penises may not get erections when they want to or may not be able to maintain them. Those with vulvas and vaginas may not naturally produce lubrication even if the person really wants to have sex. You might struggle to ejaculate or experience orgasm, or struggle with timing. Those experiences can be frustrating. We may feel shame and embarrassment around our bodies not responding the way we want them to.

Arousal non-concordance can work the other way around as well. Our bodies often respond physically to unwanted sexual stimuli, including abuse and assault. The abuse might make us feel sexually aroused, even to the point of orgasm or ejaculation. This can be very confusing and can make the trauma of sexual abuse even worse. It can feel like a betrayal by your own body. It can make you wonder if you really did want it to happen. Your body responding doesn't mean you wanted it or that the other person had permission from you to do what they did. If you want more information on this topic, I highly recommend Emily Nagoski's TED Talk titled *The Truth About Unwanted Arousal* (2018).

Recognizing the full scope of sexual abuse, including non-physical violations, is critical to understanding the impact and processing through it. Abuse isn't just about the act itself. It's also about the way it impacts your sense of self, your sense of safety, and your ability to connect with others.

Exercise 12–2:

1. What emotions and thoughts came up for you as you read through these definitions? Did anything surprise you?
2. Have you experienced anything in the above categories? If so, how did it impact you? How did you handle it? If you told others, what reactions did they have?

Consent

Sexual abuse in general is about some level of participation in sexual activity without your consent. Let's define "consent." It's more than just "yes" or "no." It's an ongoing process of mutual agreement in which each person is safe, respected, and autonomous. The *Cambridge Dictionary* (Cambridge University Press, n.d.) defines consent in general as "permission or agreement." They elaborate on the definition of the word in relation to sexual activity, explaining that it cannot be given by someone in a position where their ability to consent is impaired, whether that be because of their age, the power dynamics in the situation, or incapacitation. They also highlight that consent can be revoked at any time.

If you've ever had a medical procedure, you had to review and sign pages and pages of information that explain what's being done and how it might impact you. Scholarly references around medical informed consent highlight several elements required to give consent (Pietrzykowski & Smilowska, 2021). One is that the patient has the right to accept or refuse treatment. An additional element is that in order to be able to consent to treatment, the patient needs to understand what they're agreeing to. They need to understand the options they have and the potential risks and benefits of each.

Let's talk about how this specifically relates to sexual interactions. There are five separate elements required for sexual consent.

- Each person is equal and has a voice.
- Each person is aware of the potential risks, benefits, and consequences.
- Each person sets their own limits and honors limits set by others.
- There is no coercion or manipulation, subtle or overt, and no impairment.
- Each person can stop at any time.

Consent does not exist if there is a power imbalance that limits someone's ability to say no to any part of the interaction. Power imbalances can be due to age, authority, or dependency. For example, one of the reasons sexual relationships between teachers and students is abuse is that the student likely faces consequences if they say "no" or end the relationship. The teacher has the ability to impact their grades and their future, therefore, consent is not possible. The same type of dynamics apply to situations where individuals work with each other, but one has the power to impact job security for the other. If someone is afraid to say no, or if there are consequences that make them worried about saying no, consent isn't possible.

There are several ways this can show up in relationships where there has been betrayal. Those who have been betrayed might fear if they don't participate in sexual activity, the person who cheated might betray them again. Individuals who have betrayed might feel as if they can't say no to their significant others because they have betrayed them and now have to make it up to them. In both situations, consent is not part of the equation.

I want to be sure to state that, just like with any other piece of information, **you have the right to decide what steps you want to take and when and how you want to take them** regarding addressing any issues you identify as you read through this material. If you connect with either of the situations I just explained, or if you feel coerced to be sexual in your relationship in any way, you can choose to continue with that pattern because it feels safer for you right now or choose to figure out how to change it now. Awareness helps us to recognize that we have a choice. It doesn't tell you what the "right" choice is for you. Identifying that **you have the right to choose what you want to do with what you understand about yourself and any relationship you may be in** is foundational consent.

It's important to understand that our right to consent does not give us the right to take away someone else's ability to consent. Misrepresentation of sexual or romantic activity within a relationship removes a partner's right to choose whether or not they want to be sexually exposed to someone else. For example, if someone gives the impression or overtly states that the relationship is closed, meaning there are no sexual interactions outside of the relationship, and that isn't accurate, consent is not possible because a fully informed choice is not possible. They don't know it's happening, so they can't choose what they want to do about it.

In order for a sexual interaction or relationship to be consensual, each person needs to be aware of potential risks, benefits, and consequences. That includes possible emotional, physical, and relational outcomes. This applies to awareness of STI risks, pregnancy risks, and emotional impact. For example, if someone lies about contraceptive use, stating they are using a condom and then taking it off, or saying they're on birth control when they aren't, that is non-consensual.

Boundaries are essential to consent. Each person has the right to decide what they are and are not comfortable with at any point in the process. Agreeing to something once, or even multiple times, does not mean you have agreed to it moving forward. Being in a committed relationship does not mean you waive the right to consent to various activities. One of my favorite quotes on this topic is that consent must be freely and enthusiastically given; the absence of "no" is *not* "yes" (GlittersaurusRex, 2021).

Coercion and manipulation eliminate consent. Consent is freely given, as mentioned above. The person cannot be forced, guilted, or pressured into something. This includes overt coercion, such as threats, intimidation, or blackmail, or it can be covert, such as guilt-tripping or persistent requests. Some examples include "if you really loved me, you'd do this," or "don't be so uptight – everyone does this," or "if you don't do this, I'll find someone who will." If someone agrees under pressure, manipulation, or fear, that is not consent.

Finally, each individual has the right to change their mind at any point, for any reason. Just because they agreed to start does not mean they have to continue. This doesn't just apply when someone says "stop." It also applies if someone freezes up, pulls away, or stops responding. If enthusiastic participation stops, then the appropriate response is to check in with them rather than assuming consent still exists.

Exercise 12–3:

1. What emotions, thoughts, or memories came up for you as you read through this? If you experienced non-consensual situations and you have not already processed through them, I highly recommend getting professional help to process the emotions around them.
2. How did this change your view of consent?
3. What, if any, changes do you think might be helpful for you to make based on this? These changes might be emotions you want to process or boundaries you want to set for yourself or within a relationship.

Healing the Trauma

If you have experienced sexual trauma, it might feel like that part of you will always be broken. The wounds may feel like they are too deep to heal. Just as with other traumas, we can heal from sexual trauma. We've used tools throughout this book to heal from other types of trauma. We can use some of the same tools to heal from sexual trauma. Processing through trauma starts with identifying that it exists and sorting through what happened. It's like putting pieces of a puzzle together so you can see the full picture (what happened to you) and determine what you want to do about it moving forward. The next several sections of this book offer tools and exercises that can be used to better understand what you've gone through in your life. As we've stated previously, **you have the right to decide what steps you want to take and when and how you want to take them.** You are welcome to read through these sections and not do any of the exercises. You can do them on a more basic level. You can decide you want to dive into them. If you choose to use these exercises to identify and process through what you've gone through, make sure you have emotional support in whatever way is best for you. If you have sexual traumas in your life that have not yet been processed, I highly recommend working with a therapist if you dig into the steps we're about to talk through.

Identifying the Trauma

Grieving is an important part of that process. Often one of the first steps toward grieving is seeing the whole picture. Two tools that can be used to see the whole picture are a trauma egg specifically around sexual experiences or a sexual history timeline that includes sexual trauma.

If you've never done a trauma egg, you can find directions by doing an internet search. Most of the directions start with drawing an egg shape, then drawing smaller circles within the egg with simple pictures representing different experiences. The original trauma egg exercise was created by Marilyn Murray (2021). She doesn't use pictures, she uses brief summaries of each experience combined with emotions related to each one, the messages you got from the experience, and what you need around it. She also includes a list of positive influences, both internal and external, to help balance out the pain. Use whichever aligns better with the way you process. Trauma egg directions often have additional information included in the process. Family roles and rules may be listed as part of the exercise. To utilize the trauma egg to process sexual trauma, focus on sexual experiences rather than trauma in general. Keep in mind that anytime you use any exercise, you can alter it so it fits for you.

A sexual history timeline can be a list of your experiences or it can be a visual representation of the timeline. It can be helpful to break your life into segments, such as five-year sections. It also can be helpful to create a life events timeline to help you make sense of when various events happened. Directions for both a life events timeline and a sexual history timeline can be found at ConnectedRecoveryTraining.com, or you can search the internet and find directions.

As we discussed in Chapter 1, trauma doesn't just come from what we experience. It also comes from how others respond to what we experience. This is true for sexual trauma as well. Being shamed or blamed for sexual abuse or having your experience dismissed is unfortunately very common. Female victims of sexual abuse or assault are often blamed and asked what they were wearing or what they did to show they "wanted" it. Male victims of sexual abuse by females are frequently dismissed and told they were "lucky." LGBTQ+ victims are commonly told they should just expect it. Kink and BDSM communities often provide significant support around violations of consent, which is very helpful, particularly as responses by those outside those communities is often incredibly dismissive, saying that the abuse was obviously wanted and asked for. As you process through experiences you've gone through, also process through how others reacted to those experiences.

Sexual abuse can significantly impact our connection to ourselves and our sexuality. One way that can manifest is through carried shame. Both John Bradshaw (1988) and Pia Mellody et al. (1989) discussed the idea of "carried shame." As we discussed in Chapter 2, shame is deep feelings of unworthiness, believing "I have to be perfect, or I suck as a human being." Those who have been sexually abused frequently struggle with internalized shame as a result of what others did to them, even though the person who was abused did nothing wrong. As we talked about in the last chapter, dysfunctional systemic patterns can make that shame worse. We can be blamed for what happened or be trapped in systemic patterns that cause us to believe it was our fault, we could have controlled it, it shouldn't have impacted us the way it did, or even that the abuse made us "damaged goods." Arousal non-concordance can make those feelings of shame even worse.

It's very common to think something like "I could have done this differently" or "I should have…" This is the bargaining stage of grief, which explores "How could I have changed the story so it had a different ending." It can be empowering and healing to figure out how you would have preferred to respond and what you'd like to change in the future. It's important to recognize that identifying that you could do something different in the future doesn't mean the abuse was warranted or that you were at fault.

Making the situation even more complicated, very few human interactions are 100% abusive. Even in abusive situations, there is often some element of connection. We might feel loved or wanted at some level by the person who abused us. We might feel special because they targeted us. Grooming and manipulation frequently involve the development of emotional connection. We can feel shame about feeling connected in any way to someone who abused us. This can make us even more confused about the situation and our role in it.

It can also teach us that vulnerability and connection aren't safe. Sexual abuse objectifies the person who is abused. This may teach us that the only way to "connect" or feel loved is sex and that we will never be valued or loved as ourselves. It could also teach us that sex is the only thing about us that others want or the only way to maintain any type of connection with others. It can also teach us that sex, sexuality, and connection are about disconnected control, either being controlled or controlling others in a way that increases our belief that we aren't worthy of love and belonging. This is the opposite of healthy control, healthy boundaries, and healthy connection with ourselves, and what we desire and need.

Some relationships that include betrayal, especially those with long-term patterns of betrayal and deception, include additional elements that impact the sexuality of those who have been betrayed. Gaslighting, working to make someone believe that reality is not reality in an attempt to maintain patterns of deception, can cause us to learn that what we need, like, or want is wrong. Being ignored, rejected, or even mocked when sexual needs or desires or boundaries are expressed can teach us that we will never be loved and valued as ourselves. Sometimes those who have been betrayed are blamed for the betrayal and told that they caused it to happen by not meeting the other person's needs. These are threats; they imply that if you don't do what they want you to do, they will betray you again. This can also lead to being sexually abused or harassed by the person who has betrayed you. They may refuse to honor any boundaries you set, forcing you into interactions you don't feel comfortable with and don't want. This is abuse and often creates significant fear and shame around sexual connection, sexual boundaries, and sexual desires.

As we discussed earlier, trauma is not just harmful experiences. It is when we don't know how to protect ourselves from being hurt again in the same way. As you consider any experiences you've gone through related to sex, give yourself permission to consider different elements of them. This is not meant to create emotional pain where there isn't any. It's meant to give you time and space to believe your internal experience of the situation.

Exercise 12–4:

1. Pick either a trauma egg or trauma timeline, or pick a completely different exercise if you prefer, and review the sexual experiences you've gone through. As we've highlighted, you get to pick the level at which you want to explore this. You can always go back and explore it at a deeper level at a later point in your process. Don't force yourself to dig deeper than you are ready to dig, or deeper than your current support system is able to provide you support around. Stop if you need to. Get support as you need it.

Processing the Trauma

Once you've identified sexual experiences that were traumatic for you, trauma treatment modalities can help you process through them. There are many different types of trauma treatment modalities. The ones I use with my clients are psychodrama, somatic experiencing, post-induction therapy, EMDR, and parts work. If you connect to one particular approach, it may be helpful to find a clinician who uses that approach. If your connection and sense of safety with the clinician is more important to you that the type of approach, then the modality used may not matter as much to you as the therapist you choose to work with.

Whether or not you use additional trauma treatment modalities, I find that parts work is often an essential part of healing related to our sexual selves. One of the first questions I ask clients when we get to this stage of recovery is "what does the sexual facet of you look like?" Everyone's answer is different.

Some people picture a very specific individual. This might be connected to what they consider to be sexy and confident, as we talked about at the very beginning of Chapter 11. For example, maybe it's a cowboy like one you would find in a Louis L'Amour novel, or a character like Jessica Rabbit, or a fabulous drag queen. It might be a D&D character, a biker or biker chick in black leather, or a person dressed in an expensive suit who is in a position of power. It could include specific vulnerabilities or strengths or both. It may be an animal like a panther or a wolf or a dolphin.

Others who picture a specific individual might picture a representation of what their sexuality currently feels like having gone through their life experiences. Maybe they are broken and completely exhausted, dressed in rags. Maybe they are almost feral, terrified of connecting with others. Maybe they are silent and have learned to be invisible. Maybe they are a mouse in a maze.

It doesn't have to be an individual. It might be a scene or item. I've had several clients who pictured situations like houses in disrepair. It could be a combination of both. Perhaps you picture this part of you as an individual in a situation. Maybe this part of you is hidden away in a locked room in a basement or the corner of an attic. Maybe they're royalty in a castle in Spain or captain of a pirate ship. A clearer understanding of this part of you can help you as you process through the experiences detailed in your sexual trauma egg or timeline. This can also help to understand any abuse you went through as it provides deeper individual context.

As you sort through your story and start to understand it better, you can put the pieces together by creating an "impact letter" specifically in relation to your sexual experiences and sexual self. My version of an impact letter can be created for yourself, to yourself, to someone else, or just to have a voice. If it's to someone else, don't start by creating it in a format that you can share with them because that will likely make you filter yourself. If you want to share it with someone, you can review it later and decide if you want to share it in the format you've created it, or if you want to change it before sharing it. The initial version is for you.

Also, this is your story, and you get to tell it your way. While the term "impact letter" usually implies a written form of communication, you can use whatever format you want. You can write it as a letter. You can write it as a story. You can write a poem. You can create a visual representation of it, such as a sculpture or a painting or a collage. You can create a music playlist that represents what it was like to go through your experiences. For some people, the timeline or trauma egg is their version of the impact letter around this part of their lives.

If you consider creating an "impact letter," make sure you set up whatever steps you need to make it safe for you to create. If you choose a written format and use an electronic device to write it, password protect it. Use a password you don't usually use and share it with someone you trust, such as your therapist or someone in your support system, in case you forget it. If you physically write something or create a visual representation, find a place to store it that feels safe for you. It will be difficult to be fully honest in the process if someone else might be able to access it without your permission.

Exercise 12–5:

1. Stop and consider what the sexual facet of you looks like. What did you resonate with and what came to mind?
2. Using whatever format works best for you, create something that represents that part. You might write a description of them, draw a picture, create a collage, create a playlist, etc.
3. Consider the experiences you listed as part of your trauma egg or trauma timeline. Did those happen to the sexual facet of you or another part of you? How does that impact your understanding of what you experienced?
4. Consider the format that would work best to put your story together (create an "impact letter"). Determine what steps you would like to take at this time around that. Make sure to get emotional support as needed.

Super Short Summary:

Sexual abuse refers to any non-consensual act or behavior imposed on an individual, regardless of the relationship between the individuals involved. Consent is a combination of agreement and knowledge. Our right to consent does not give us the right to take away someone else's ability to consent. It's important to process through any abuse we've experienced. Trauma treatment is often necessary to process through sexual abuse.

Chapter Questions:

1. What did you connect to the most in this chapter?
2. What steps are you taking to apply this material to your life?

13

Boundaries
Replace, Reclaim, and Redefine

Sorting through the experiences you've gone through and identifying the trauma and pain connected to them is heavy and can leave us feeling as though everything we've gone through has been tainted and nothing is safe. You may have already felt that going into Chapter 12 due to whatever you experienced that led you to read this book, although the last chapter may have left you feeling heavier. Maybe the work we did in the last chapter left you feeling lighter. Perhaps it was validating to give voice to the pain you've experienced.

Whatever you experienced as you sorted through the work around identifying and processing traumatic experiences you've gone through related to sexuality, moving into acceptance requires safety. As we've discussed throughout this book, safety requires boundaries. The boundaries component of late recovery focuses on replacing, reclaiming, and redefining parts of ourselves and our lives in relation to the deepest connection to ourselves. Setting clear boundaries helps us create safety and regain autonomy individually and relationally as it relates to our bodies, needs, and desires. Going through the steps in this chapter can help us reset our sexual boundaries in a way that aligns with who we are and who we want to become. Using the Hierarchy of Needs as a reference, it provides the foundation of safety, allowing us the freedom to focus on deepening connection to ourselves and others, build our confidence, and eventually relax and explore this aspect of ourselves and our connection with others. We're moving from survival into growth.

There are four steps to this part of the process: recognize, replace, reclaim, and redefine. We recognize the aspects of our sexuality and connection to sexual interactions with self and others around which we still have unwanted pain and triggers, determine which of those we want to replace and how to replace them, consider which we want to reclaim, and which we need to redefine in order to move toward who we want to be and how we want to show up for ourselves and others.

Recognize

The first step of this process is identifying unwanted pain points and triggers, or aspects that feel out of alignment with ourselves. The work we did in the last chapter often helps to make these more obvious. These can be triggers, responses in our bodies, unwanted patterns that cause disconnection, or even inherited or imposed beliefs.

DOI: 10.4324/9781003623359-17

As we go through these steps, it's important to separate shame from the process. As we discussed in Chapter 2, shame prevents us from being able to move forward as it makes us believe that whatever we're feeling is inherently wrong, that we are broken or don't have the right to feel the emotions we feel or set the boundaries we need. Using the same tools we discussed earlier, if shame comes up as you go through this step, stop and separate the shame from the emotion or need so you can process through each because both will give you information.

Throughout this book, we've talked through understanding ourselves better. In Chapter 2 we discussed our strengths, weaknesses, fears, abilities, and potential. In Chapter 7 we discussed family roles and rules. In Chapter 12, we explored sexual trauma. Each of these provides context for why we feel what we feel and think what we think. It makes sense. In Chapter 10 we discussed empathy for self. Empathy for self is crucial as we move through this step.

This step invites curiosity and compassion, allowing us to acknowledge unwanted pain points and triggers without judgment, creating a space for healing and connection. Struggles in this area are not a personal failing, but a response to past experiences. Identifying what is causing us unwanted discomfort, disconnection, or distress gives us the opportunity to create a roadmap for change, offering insights into what we need to replace, reclaim, and redefine.

Triggers

Let's start by considering triggers. As a reminder, triggers are terror, meaning automatic responses by our nervous system to things that have previously harmed us. They send us messages that we need to protect ourselves. As we discussed in Chapter 3, triggers can show up in different areas. They might be related to certain words or phrases. Maybe we have triggers around certain people, places, or things. Perhaps we have triggers around emotions, specific physical activities, or specific social interactions.

Exercise 13–1:

1. What triggers you? Consider words, phrases, people, places, things, emotions, physical activities, and social interactions.
2. Did any shame come up for you as you considered your triggers? If so, separate the shame from the emotion and process both. Use the Processing Shame Worksheet (available at ConnectedRecoveryTraining.com) if needed.

Physical and Emotional Disconnection

Triggers aren't the only area we need to consider. There may also be responses in our bodies that are different from what we want them to be. Remembering our conversation in Chapter 12 about arousal non-concordance, give yourself time and space to process any physical responses you may have had that you didn't want to have. Take that a step further and consider the situation that produced that response in you. These may highlight areas we need additional boundaries around in order to feel safe enough to connect with ourselves and others.

Be curious about how your body reacts to different situations. Do you feel unwanted tension or dissociation? Do you shut down? Do you chameleon? I'll take a minute to describe the term. I use that word as a verb to describe shifting into something to try and match the people and situations we are connected to, rather than staying ourselves. Some level of chameleoning is natural and helpful. For example, there are elements of me that show up differently as a therapist versus a mother versus a friend versus a wife, but staying true to myself and connected to myself in each role is important.

Imbalanced or extreme chameleoning disconnects us from ourselves. In relation to sexuality, sometimes this is related to cycles of avoidance, unwanted patterns of hypersexuality, or emotional disconnection or intensity that may stem from past trauma. Other times, those elements may not be present or may be unrelated to chameleoning. The deeper we get into this work, the more individual the work becomes. Consider what you connect to and what you disconnect to as we talk through these topics. Again, we're looking at these elements with curiosity and compassion. If shame comes up, meaning if you start judging yourself for what you're recognizing, take a step back, separate the shame from the emotion or thought, and process each so you have the information from each as you move forward.

These elements can show up as avoiding touch, or not allowing ourselves to feel or acknowledge attraction, or experience connection due to unwanted fear or discomfort. These responses make sense in the context of what you've experienced in the past or in the context of current patterns related to sexuality. This isn't about shaming yourself for developing those responses, it's about identifying what you would like to be different as you move forward.

Exercise 13–2:

1. Are there times you avoid sexual connection as a way to numb or avoid emotions?
2. Do you connect with the term "chameleon" in relation to sexuality? Why or why not?

Incongruent Hypersexuality

Perhaps you go to the other extreme of the continuum, turning to incongruent hypersexuality. This may be related to using sexual connection to numb or soothe yourself in disconnecting and incongruent ways. It could also be related to using sexual connection or activity for external validation in an unbalanced way. We're looking for lack of balance in validation, not shifting to dismissing needs and wants. There is nothing wrong with wanting to feel wanted, desired, or loved. It can become imbalanced when we don't have foundational connection with ourselves. In those cases, it can feel like desperation and no matter how much validation we get, it's not enough. It can lead to experiencing sexual connection as mechanical, unfulfilling, and disconnecting.

Incongruent hypersexuality might also be related to performative sex. Performative sex is participating in sexual activity based on what someone else wants at the expense of your needs and wants. As we've talked about throughout this book, moderate and balanced incorporation of each factor is healthy. In this case, considering what others we are connected to want or need is important. This becomes unhealthy when we ignore our needs or wants and ignore our boundaries, creating a lack of safety for ourselves, which makes it very difficult to work toward connection, confidence, and joy.

Exercise 13–3:

1. Have you experienced incongruent hypersexuality? If so, was it related to emotional numbing or performative sex?

Inherited or Imposed Beliefs

We talked about the connection between shame and sexuality in the last chapter and the sexual trauma egg or timeline, along with the impact letter helped to identify shame-based messages, inherited or imposed beliefs, that may have been instilled in us by the families, societal groups, or cultural groups we have been or are currently connected to. These messages might be related to sexual acts, expression, or orientation, relational orientation, intimacy, or self-worth. They may have taught shame or fear and create confusion about our sexuality.

We may have been taught that sex is dirty, wrong, or shameful. Perhaps we were taught that we aren't allowed to enjoy it, or that we can only enjoy certain things. We might have been taught that we aren't allowed to say no. We might believe that sexual connection always has to be spontaneous, perfect, and passionate, or we believe that sexual connection exists only for procreation. Very commonly we are taught that if we struggle with anything related to sexual connection, there is something wrong with us.

Exercise 13–4:

1. What messages did you receive about sex growing up?
2. Are there beliefs you hold about sexuality that cause you to feel shame or disregard your emotions, needs, and desires? If so, what are they?
3. Based on external influences rather than your own preferences, do you feel you "should" like or dislike certain sexual experiences? If so, what?

Replace

Now that we've compiled our lists of what is causing harm in our sexual connection with ourselves and others, the next step is to determine if we want to replace, reclaim, or redefine each element. Let's start with replace.

Replace is the healthy, balanced version of avoidance. It's about empowered choice, not about numbing or escaping. This step allows us to remove unnecessary triggers and unwanted pain points that interfere with our healing and our connection to ourselves and others. It helps us to create boundaries that build a foundation for new, intentional experiences that feel safe and affirming. There are three distinct areas this can be helpful in: words and language, items, and situations.

Words and Language

Words hold power. Language can trigger pain or promote healing. Specific sexual terms, such as pet names, certain terms, slang words, unwanted degrading language, etc. can emotionally and mentally transport us back to a situational or emotional memory that push on our "brakes" instead of our "accelerators." In some cases, we may want to reclaim these. In others, we would prefer to replace them. It can be difficult to give ourselves permission to set boundaries in this area. If you are in a relationship and it's relationally safe, I recommend talking within your relationship about what you're doing and why you're doing it. I recommend phrases like "I prefer not to use [word] in sexual communication. Can we use [alternative] instead?" or "[Word] takes me out of the experience. Can we come up with different language that helps me stay more connected to the experience?"

Don't shame yourself or others about the words that you connect with or disconnect with. You are working to maximize the potential for connection. Remember way back in the introduction when we talked about bucket-fillers? This is the same tool. Find words and phrases that feel empowering, connecting, and safe for you. At the very least, look for words and phrases that are neutral rather than triggering or uncomfortable.

Keep in mind that these will be different for each person and each relationship. While one person might be triggered by degrading language, another might be turned on by it. That's why I used the word "unwanted" in the first paragraph of this section. If what turns one person on triggers another person in a relationship, consider interactions that each person feels safe with while sorting through how to balance differing desires and needs. A sex therapist can help with this part of the process. If there has been betrayal in the relationship, look for a sex therapist with a betrayal-sensitive approach.

Exercise 13–5:

1. What words or phrases are triggering or disconnecting for you? Which would you like to replace and which would you like to reclaim?
2. If you are in a relationship, do you feel emotionally safe to have a relational conversation about changing those words or phrases? If not, are there steps you could take that would make you feel safer to have that conversation?
3. How might you know if you need to stop the conversation? What support might you need if you have to take that step?

Items

Physical objects, sounds, or sensory experiences often hold emotional weight. We considered how we could get joy from connecting with each of our senses in the bucket-fillers part of the introduction. Each of our senses can trigger us as well. Something as simple as a song, perfume, or piece of clothing may mentally and emotionally connect you to past trauma, shame, or unwanted pain. For example, a song that either you remember from a past event or that describes emotions or situations similar to something you went through might trigger a memory or emotion. Clothing might feel emotionally or physically restrictive, disempowering, or might trigger a memory. Scents and tastes can remind us of experiences we've gone through as well.

As with words and language, you can choose if you want to replace those or reclaim them. For those you want to replace, find new, intentionally chosen items that make you feel safe and confident, or at the very least, neutral. What are you comfortable with? What do you like? Give yourself permission to learn who you are.

I've had clients get rid of clothing, redesign bedrooms or other rooms in their homes, and find new soaps, lotions, shampoo, perfume, or cologne. Some change their style completely, others might replace specific items. Changing your style completely might be helpful if your former style no longer aligns with who you feel you are or if you feel your former style was more about being who someone else wanted you to be.

Exercise 13–6:

1. What items trigger unwanted painful emotions for you? Which would you like to reclaim and which would you like to replace?
2. What might you be able to replace those items with that would feel empowering to you? If empowerment does not seem possible at the moment, what might you replace them with that would feel neutral?

Situations

As with words, language, and items, certain places, interactions, or even sexual positions may be tied to unwanted painful memories or produce a trigger response. This might apply to specific restaurants, hotels, stores, or other specific locations. It might apply to a general type of location, like beaches or pools or concerts. It could be specific types of sexual interactions or specific sexual positions.

Just like each of the other categories, these situations might be ones you want to reclaim. We'll explain how to reclaim parts of ourselves and our lives in the next section of this chapter. Also, recognize that deciding to replace something can be a temporary choice. You might need to replace it now but want to consider reclaiming it in the future. That's ok. You get to decide what's right for you.

Sometimes one person in a relationship wants to replace something and another feels it is important to reclaim it. Finding the right language around this conversation can be difficult, but it's an important step. Often if someone wants to replace something, it means they can't imagine ever feeling safe with it again, and it's not uncommon for those emotions to be expressed as "I am never, ever, ever, doing this again." It may be accurate that the individual will never feel safe with it again and that's ok if they never do. There are ways to work through whatever each person needs. I've found it's more helpful to say something like "I know this is important to you, but as of right now, I can't imagine how I would ever feel safe with it again. Could we please replace it for now?" That language gives each person more time to advocate for what they need and want and to process the emotions connected to it. You don't have to know what you'll need or want for the rest of your life. You just need to know what you need for now.

Replacing situations might include finding new restaurants to visit. It might mean you prefer to vacation to the mountains instead of the beach or avoid specific cities or areas. It might include eliminating sexual positions or types of sexual interactions, such as oral sex. As we'll talk about in the next two chapters, there are lots of ways to connect sexually. Referring to Chapter 6, remember that often we mislabel a potential solution that might be one way to meet a need as the "need." There may be specific solutions that are really, really important to you, and processing through that is critical. In situations where one person's boundaries seem to conflict with another person's needs, I recommend you consider the foundational need and consider the cost of what you're asking for. You get to decide what is most important to you. At the same time, you don't get to tell someone else that they have to do something they don't want to do. We discussed that concept when we explained consent in Chapter 12.

Exercise 13–7:

1. What locations or sexual positions or interactions currently trigger unwanted emotional pain for you? Which would you like to reclaim and which would you like to replace?
2. What boundaries related to locations might be helpful for you as you move forward in this area? What boundaries related to sexual interactions might be helpful for you?

Reclaim

Reclaiming is about actively working to take back yourself, your body, your life, and your identity. It helps you to regain things that were lost, connection that was suppressed, and areas of your life that the trauma you went through distorted or stole. Reclaiming is about actively choosing what belongs to you and what you want to claim back. It helps to empower you and move you toward deeper authentic connection with yourself and others.

We can reclaim words and language, clothing or even styles of clothing, music, sensory triggers, locations, interactions, and sexual expression or positions. Reclaiming starts with identifying that something has caused us unwanted pain or triggers us, but we want to do the work to be able to connect to it again.

> **Exercise 13–8:**
>
> 1. Your answers from the exercises in the previous section include listing what you would like to reclaim. Go through those answers and create a list of the things you want to reclaim for yourself.
> 2. Consider your list and pick one to focus on as we go through the rest of this section.

Be aware that there may be items on the list that you know you want to reclaim at some point, but it doesn't feel feasible right now. That's ok. Knowing you want to reclaim them at some point puts them on your radar and you can take those steps when you're ready to do so.

The first step to reclaiming something is to understand what it used to mean to you or what you got from it before the experiences you went through tainted it. In some cases, it's not directly about whatever it is you're claiming back, it's about what the trigger is costing you. For example, you might be triggered by a location, such as Vegas. You may not necessarily care if you ever go to Vegas again or not, but perhaps there's a conference you regularly go to that is held in Vegas and the trigger related to the city is preventing you from enjoying the conference. In this case, what was stolen from you is the ability to enjoy the conference. Think about what you're working on reclaiming. What are you claiming back?

Understanding what you're specifically focused on helps you as you move to the next step, which is processing through the pain that took it from you. This processing is similar to a highly focused impact letter in that you're exploring what happened and how it impacted you. Utilize whatever format works best for you. Often my clients process the pain verbally in a session, sometimes using trauma treatment modalities such as somatic experiencing, psychodrama, or EMDR.

Once you understand this part of your story, the next step is to develop a plan of action. I use the term "bookending" for this part of the process. Picture a set of bookends. One is at the beginning of the set, and one holds up the end. The books are propped up in the middle. Using bookending, we review the situation before going into it, deciding how we want to navigate it. Throughout the experience, we check in regularly and determine if we need to activate any of the potential supports we put in place. At the end, we review how it went, determine what went well and why, along with what we'd like to change in similar situations in the future and if there's anything we need to process from the experience.

We also determine where potential triggers might be. We're deliberately incorporating what we want to take back. Think about what you might want to include that would help you reclaim it.

For example, if your birthday is now a painful reminder to you of a trauma you went through or something that was done to you, you might plan something special for that day, incorporating several close friends. Figure out the steps that are right for you. It might feel right for you to have a few close friends over and talk about the pain connected to your birthday. Or it might feel right for you to throw a big party and deliberately work to feel the joy you've been missing. Or it might feel right to plan a special trip, going somewhere you've always wanted to go or doing something you've always wanted to do. The steps we take to reclaim something are very individual and will likely differ dramatically depending on what you're claiming back.

As you're creating whatever plan is right for you, make sure to incorporate how you will address triggers if they come up. Will you pause and process through the trigger? Or would it fit better for you to flip it off or laugh in its face? Who might be able to support you as you take these steps?

After developing your plan, put it into action. Check in with yourself throughout the process. Afterwards, review your experience. What went well and what would you like to have done differently? Do you need to process anything that came up for you?

The final step is looking back at what you're reclaiming. Do you have it back? If not, go through and repeat the steps. Sometimes we claim things back in layers. If you don't feel like you're making progress with a specific thing, I recommend processing it with your therapist and working to see why you are stuck. As we've discussed multiple times, honor what you're feeling. If there is an emotional wall, don't try to knock it down. Figure out why the wall is there and what message it's sending you. We build walls for a reason. Sometimes figuring out why they are there gives you the key you need to get to the other side. Other times we figure out that we need the wall there and decide where to go from there. Sometimes we are able to process through it and take it down brick by brick.

Exercise 13–9:

1. What came up for you as you considered going through this process? What did you connect with? What did you disconnect with?
2. What did you learn about yourself? How do you think this will impact you moving forward?

Redefine

After recognizing, replacing, and reclaiming, we move on to redefining. Redefining in this section refers to specific things, such as words or language, items, or situations. Redefining sexuality on your terms is the next chapter. This section focuses on actively reshaping words, items, and situations so they align with your healing, identity, and personal empowerment. Replacing removes triggers, reclaiming restores autonomy, and redefining allows us to take ownership of our experience related to specific things. Redefining means you, and only you, get to determine what something means for you going forward. This step helps us to reshape narratives and craft a personal, empowered relationship with things that were tainted by our experiences.

While replacing is fairly straightforward, understanding the difference between reclaiming and redefining can be difficult. The two are interconnected but they play different roles. Reclaiming is about taking back what was lost, stolen, or tainted. It's about ownership and autonomy. Redefining is about reshaping meaning to align with who you are and who you want to become. It's about creating new personal truths.

Words and Language

As we've mentioned, words and language have power. While there are some words that can be replaced, and others that we can reclaim, there are some that need to be redefined. Some of those are words that give us permission to connect to ourselves, others are ones that have been used as weapons against us.

Words that give us permission to connect with ourselves and our experiences include words like sensual, arousal, fantasy, desire, need, want, attraction, and passion. These may have also been used as sources of shame or suppression. When redefined, they give us permission to create an empowered relationship with ourselves and our experiences.

Let's use sensuality as an example. It's not about performance or what others think of you. It doesn't mean you have to respond in any specific way. At its core, the word sensuality refers to connecting to yourself and your experience using your senses. Think about an experience that you connect to using multiple senses. For example, standing on the beach. One of my favorite beaches is Seven Mile Beach on Grand Cayman. When I think about being there, I can almost hear the waves lapping on the shore, the sound of the birds and voices of others at the beach in the distance. I can almost feel the warmth of the sun combined with the cooler feeling of the water and the soft sand beneath. I can almost smell the salt in the air from the water and taste the spray from the waves that lingers in the air. And I can almost see the combination of the beautiful blue of the Caribbean water and the light tan of the sand. I can picture watching the sun set over the water and seeing the pinks and purples of the sky. This is a much deeper description and experience than saying I stood on the beach. The difference between those two descriptions, the first with all the sense-related details, and the second comprised of five basic words, is the difference between the experience you can have when you give yourself permission to connect to your senses and that when you don't. Redefining the word sensual gives us permission to experience.

Each of the words I listed gives us a different type of permission to connect with ourselves and our lives. Arousal gives us permission to feel. It's about sensing the energy within us. Fantasy is the permission to imagine. It allows us to experiment with ideas, desires, and emotions. Desire is permission to want. It helps us understand what we want and how we want it. Need is permission to prioritize ourselves. As we discussed in Chapter 6, it is not weakness, it's essential. Want is permission to choose. It's about identifying personal preferences. Attraction is permission to feel drawn to something. This might be people, ideas, or experiences. Passion is permission to fully engage. It helps us connect with experiences, relationships, and pursuits that set our soul on fire. Redefining these words gives us permission to feel, explore, and connect with ourselves and our experiences. They help us build a relationship with ourselves founded in choice, authenticity, confidence, and joy.

The second type of words we can reclaim are those used as weapons against us. The phrase for this is linguistic resistance. There are many examples of this in society. The word "queer" was originally a slur. It has been reclaimed by the LGBTQ+ community and is now an inclusive term that represents fluidity and self-acceptance outside of societal and cultural norms related to gender, orientation, and sexuality. Two other well-known examples are "nerd" and "geek." When I was growing up, these words were used to make fun of those who were interested in studying or technology. They are now often used as badges of honor.

There are many other examples. Linguistic resistance takes power away from those who have oppressed others and returns it to the people the words were used against. It allows us to define ourselves on our own terms. We redefine words by identifying the power they currently have for us, attaching a new meaning to it, and then reinforcing that new meaning in an empowered way.

In my experience, each of us has one or two specific words that are most painful for us. One of the most common words my female clients have listed is "bitch." One of the group activities I've done with group where the members were female is an art therapy project where they embraced their inner "bitch." We'd listen to songs that used the word in a way they felt empowered by, talk about what the word meant to each of us and how it had been used in our lives, then shift into talking about the power behind it and how we wanted to harness that power.

Exercise 13–10:

1. Which of the words that give us permission did you most connect to? Why?
2. Take a minute and consider the words that are most painful for you. Pick one. Consider the power it has had for you and how it's been used as a weapon against you. Use art (paint a picture, create a sculpture, create a collage), language (write a poem), music (find one specific song or create a playlist), or another medium to identify the power behind it and how you are going to connect to that power.

Items

As we talked about earlier in this chapter, certain items, like clothing, music, scents, or specific objects, can be tied to memories that trigger you or cause you unwanted pain. Redefining these items means looking at the emotional connection you have to them and transforming their meaning so they align with who you are and who you want to be. It's about changing the way we perceive, interact with, or experience objects. It's reshaping our relationship with them, and in doing so, changing our relationship with ourselves.

This process is similar to the one we just talked about in relation to linguistic resistance, although this applies those tools to specific items rather than words. Let's use high heels as an example. High heels are one of the most symbolically charged fashion items in modern culture. They are often associated with male approval, sexualization, or femininity standards. If you want to wear heels, redefining high heels means choosing what they mean for you rather than accepting the meanings imposed by others. Instead of seeing heels as something you "have to wear" or as something that makes other people think you are sexy, you can reclaim them as a source of confidence, personal power, and self-expression. Or maybe you figure out that you don't actually want to wear them, you were only wearing them because you felt like you were supposed to, so you reject them entirely in favor of something that aligns better with your values.

Redefining deepens our connection to ourselves, allowing us to honor what we really want and how we want to feel. It increases our ability to choose. Referring to the example above, redefining heels means you have a greater ability to choose how they fit into your life. You can wear them with intention, feeling the empowerment and confidence you get from them. You can reject them completely and create comfort and confidence for yourself by choosing something else. And you can alternate, depending on what makes you feel more empowered in the moment.

To redefine an item, start by recognizing the meaning the item currently has to you. What is your connection to it? What emotions come up for you around it? Work to identify historical or personal meanings that don't align with who you are and who you want to be. As you work through this step, you may also identify meanings that you want to strengthen. Decide what you want the item to symbolize for you. How can it empower you? Do you want to stay connected with it or replace it with something else? Once you redefine what it means to you, you can choose to use it in a way that connects you with yourself.

Exercise 13–11:

1. What items either cause you unwanted pain, trigger you, or carry a meaning you no longer connect to?
2. What messages, emotions, and memories are connected to those items? Which would you like to keep, and which would you like to change?
3. How can you redefine them to empower yourself and better represent who you are and who you want to be?

Situations

Redefining situations is about changing the way we interpret, engage with, and internalize experiences. It's how we reshape their meaning in a way that aligns with our growth and healing. Sometimes it's difficult to understand the difference between redefining and reclaiming. Reclaiming is about taking back something that was lost, stolen, or tainted, but redefining is about reshaping the experience completely, creating a new framework for how we engage with it on our own terms. It's about shifting our perspective and transforming the situation into a way that provides purpose, meaning, and an opportunity for growth. Redefining is not about pretending things didn't happen. It's about changing how they live inside of us.

This is closely aligned with the last two stages of grief that we talked about in Chapter 2 – making meaning and acceptance. These stages focus on transformation and resolution. They involve understanding what happened and reshaping its impact on us. Making meaning involves actively choosing what we are going to do with what happened to us. Acceptance is about finding peace and moving forward, creating a new relationship with our experiences so they no longer hold power over us.

Redefining situations allows us to reframe unwanted pain as a source of wisdom. Not because we are ok with what was done, but because we are actively deciding how we want to grow from it. It shifts our grief and pain from passive to active. It allows us to detach from needing the past to be different, releasing old narratives, and finding a way to integrate our unwanted pain into peace. It defines our experiences as chapters, or even a section in a chapter, rather than our whole book or how our story ends. It allows for peace without denying the impact of the situation. It shifts into focusing on what is possible rather than what was lost.

Redefining helps us identify boundaries we need as we move forward, building safety and preventing future harm. When we redefine situations, we don't just change how we think and feel about the past, we also change how we engage with similar situations in the future. It helps us clarify our boundaries, needs, and expectations.

Let's use growing up in an abusive family as an example. Before we delve into this example, recognize that it is very difficult to redefine abusive situations while you are still in them. This connects to the material we covered in the introduction and in all of Phase 1. You have to be safe before you can move on to the higher stages of the Hierarchy of Needs. Redefining is related to Self-Actualization, which is the fourth level of the Hierarchy of Needs. Usually we need to have our basic needs met, have foundational safety in our lives and in our connection with others, and have support in order to have the foundation to redefine unwanted pain we've experienced.

Let's get back to our example. Childhood abuse is one of the most deeply impactful experiences a person can go through. It often shapes our identity, belief about our self-worth, the way we connect with others, and the way we connect with ourselves, and those influences can last throughout adulthood if not addressed. Redefining an experience like childhood abuse is not rewriting the story. It doesn't erase what you went through. Instead, it changes the way we see ourselves having lived through it. It changes the meaning we assign to it. It changes how it influences our future, our relationship with ourselves and with others, and our healing.

The first step to redefining an experience like this is identifying the narratives that were formed as a result. These likely became faulty core beliefs, which we discussed in Chapter 2. Maybe you learned that you weren't worthy of being loved. Maybe you learned you were too much or not enough. Maybe you learned you can never trust anyone. Whatever messages you internalized from those experiences, those messages were never true. They were imposed by the actions of others and reinforced by shame, secrecy, and dysfunction.

Once you've identified the narratives, the next step is to challenge them. Consider if the meaning you've ascribed to them is accurate or helpful. How much of the situation did you have the power to control? How much of what was said would you think was accurate if it was said to a friend? How much aligns with your understanding of your current self and the messages you hear from those who love you and are currently connected to you in meaningful ways?

Finally, create a new, empowering definition. Choose a new way to see its impact on your life. Factor in the changes you've made, the work you've done, who you are now, and who you are becoming. This doesn't diminish or dismiss the pain you went through. It allows you to redefine how this pain will impact your future. Consider your strengths and abilities as we talked about in Chapter 2. Consider the tools you've developed. Instead of "I can't trust anyone," perhaps your truth is now "I was really hurt by what I went through. I couldn't trust anyone. Now I see that it was their dysfunction, not who I am. I have the tools to build healthy relationships, set boundaries, and foster connection with myself and others."

Exercise 13–12:

1. Think about the situations you've gone through. Which of those would you like to define?
2. How did those experiences teach you to view yourself?
3. What do you want to learn from them? How do you want to move forward?

Super Short Summary:

Setting clear boundaries for ourselves helps us create safety and regain autonomy and move from survival into growth. There are four steps to this part of the process: recognize, replace, reclaim, and redefine. Recognizing involves identifying the aspects of our sexuality and connection to sexual interactions with self and others around which we still have unwanted pain and triggers, including words and language, items, and situations. We can then choose which we want to replace, which we want to reclaim, and which we want to redefine.

Chapter Questions:

1. What did you connect to the most in this chapter?
2. What steps are you taking to apply this material to your life?

14

Communication

Self-Exploration

The communication component of late recovery focuses on communicating with yourself and learning what you like and don't like, emotionally and physically. Throughout this book, we've taken steps that help you to get to know yourself better. This whole process is about getting to know yourself, connecting to who you are, and helping you heal from what you've gone through and become fully yourself. We've dug into this at various levels. For example, in the introduction, we considered sensory bucket-fillers, a basic level of connecting to yourself by figuring out what you like to taste, smell, see, hear, and feel. In Chapter 2, we explored defining yourself and understanding your strengths and weaknesses, including resentments, fears, abilities, accomplishments, and potential. Chapter 7 considered the patterns you experienced and how they shaped who you've become. Chapter 11 had you consider what sexy means to you and what deep connection with yourself in a way that makes you feel confident and whole might look like. In the last chapter we discussed reclaiming parts of your life and redefining others, addressing the trauma, pain, and dysfunction that may have colored your deepest connection to yourself.

By the time we get to this step in the process, it may feel like all that's left of your sexuality is a grain of sand, surrounded by blackness. But hopefully the unwanted pain and trauma and faulty core beliefs and dysfunction have been addressed to the point that they no longer have the power to eat away at you and destroy you. Seeing yourself, understanding yourself, is the first step toward rebuilding your sexual world in a way that brings you joy and connection.

This chapter is about rediscovering yourself. Or perhaps discovering yourself for the very first time. This chapter focuses on helping you explore who you are and what you want, free from shame, fear, or imposed expectations. Self-exploration is not about "fixing" yourself. It's about getting to know yourself and believing your internal experience at multiple levels. Understanding your likes and dislikes, your strengths and vulnerabilities, your emotions, boundaries, and values. It's about creating an empowered relationship with your body, your emotions, and your authentic self. It's about developing confidence so you can experience joy. "Confidence is knowing what's true. Joy is loving what's true" (Nagoski, 2016).

Self-exploration can be divided into three domains: emotional, physical, and arousal. Emotional exploration involves identifying and honoring your emotions, understanding the messages they carry, and creating space for yourself to process them without judgment.

DOI: 10.4324/9781003623359-18

Physical exploration includes becoming familiar with your body in a way you are comfortable with, which is why we address the emotional aspect first. Physical exploration is not about forced masturbation or sexual interactions. It's about creating a sense of safety, curiosity, and acceptance within your own skin. Exploring the arousal domain connects emotional and physical domains, helping you to understand what you want and how you want it. This includes understanding what feels safe for you, what excites you, and what aligns with your values and sense of self.

Emotional Exploration

As we've discussed throughout this book, emotions are not random, and they give us very valuable information and help connect us to ourselves and others. We've worked through how to identify and process your emotions, factoring them into the choices you make and the boundaries you set. In general, emotions are often dismissed, minimized, or misunderstood. Emotions connected to sexuality are even more likely to be suppressed.

The last two chapters helped to work through some of the instigating factors that repress emotions related to sexuality. As we talked about earlier, pleasure, desire, and arousal are frequently framed as shameful, dirty, or inappropriate. The internalized shame around sex and sexuality often leads to confusion about what you truly want, or even avoidance of the whole topic.

Emotional suppression, due to societal conditioning, cultural messaging, or trauma, disconnects us from ourselves and others. Your emotions are valid, important, and a critical part of connection. Emotional exploration is not about forcing yourself to feel and connect differently overnight. It's about gradually creating space for your emotions in a way that fosters understanding, self-compassion and empathy, compassion and empathy for others, and personal empowerment.

It's important to start from a place of curiosity rather than judgment. If you feel judgment coming into the equation, step back and consider the judgment with curiosity as well. Where did it come from? Whose voice is it? Why is it showing up? What message is it trying to send you? Why is it worried about you looking at whatever it is you're working to understand? What is it afraid of? Judgment is almost always founded in fear. Once you understand the judgment better, you can figure out what you need to do with the information it gave you.

At its core, sexuality is about connection with yourself. It's about understanding yourself at the deepest level through emotional awareness, self-acceptance, and a willingness to explore your desires, fears, and vulnerabilities without judgment. As we've stated multiple times throughout the last several chapters, **you get to process through this at your own speed.** You get to decide what steps are right for you and when you want to take them. The concepts and tools provided are here when you're ready to explore them.

Your sexuality is an extension of your inner world. Your inner world includes the way you love, connect, experience pleasure, and process emotions. Understanding your sexuality at an emotional level means moving beyond doing what you think you "should," liking what you think you "should," being who you think you "should." Authentic sexuality is engaging in what genuinely aligns with your emotions, values, and desires.

Shame is often a significant barrier, as we've talked about. In this case, shame manifests as feeling that sexual desires, thoughts, or experiences are "wrong" or "dirty." This might be related to sex in general or might apply to specific interests or experiences. It may be related to internalized societal scripts about what sexuality "should" look like rather than focusing on what feels right personally. If there is trauma connected to those, or if you struggle to listen to their message and process through it, I recommend you work with a therapist to process through that experience or faulty core belief.

There may also be a lot of fear related to this topic that is not shame-based. Fear of vulnerability is common, especially if you've been hurt in the past. The deeper we work to know ourselves, the deeper it hurts when we are rejected or judged or unwanted. This is where connection to self comes into play, although it goes hand in hand with having a system that supports you. The work we've done to strengthen your connection to yourself helps provide a foundation that allows you to move toward openness as you know you won't reject yourself and you know you have connection with those around you, so you won't be abandoned as you go through this process, even when it is difficult. Reconnecting emotionally with your sexuality means embracing it as a valid and beautiful part of who you are. It requires deep self-awareness and emotional courage. As we move forward with these steps, it's often helpful to connect it with the work we did in Chapter 12 around the sexual facet of you.

Exercise 14–1:

1. Review the parts work we did in Chapter 12. What represents the sexual facet of you?
2. Consider the work you did in Chapter 13. Did that clarify any aspect of this part of you? If so, what?
3. Does that part of you look the same as it did when you originally did the exercise? If not, what's changed? Why did it change?

Identifying Your Emotions

There are three questions that can help you with emotional exploration. The first is "What emotions arise when I think about my sexuality?" It's often a combination of several. Maybe you feel excited but scared about connecting to yourself at that level or scared about being rejected if you do. Perhaps you're more curious. Maybe you feel guilt or grief around things that you've done or things that have happened to you. Maybe it's difficult to feel anything and you feel numb. Maybe you feel joy at finally being able to consider this aspect of yourself. As we mentioned earlier, if shame comes up at any point in this process, separate it from the emotion and process why you're feeling it, where it comes from, and what message it's trying to send you.

The next question to consider is "Have I been taught or have I learned that certain emotions around sex are 'bad' or 'wrong'?" Are there ways you aren't allowed to feel, either because of something you were taught by others or something you learned as a result of experiences you went through? This question focuses on internal beliefs about emotions related to sexuality. It helps you explore how you judge your own emotions and whether you allow yourself to feel and express them. It addresses how you interpret and regulate feelings like desire, excitement, passion, vulnerability, or fear. Do you feel like it's ok to feel desire or pleasure? Are there specific rules about what you're allowed to feel and when and how you're allowed to feel it?

It's often helpful to consider if there are aspects of your sexuality that you feel are "unnatural" or "deviant" or "off-limits." This may apply to certain positions or sex acts, ways of presenting yourself you feel would be sexy, but are at odds with what you believe is "ok" to want. In some cases, this may be enjoying sex in general. It might be anything other than heterosexual sex using missionary position. It may be that those words themselves are ones you connect with sexually and they feel empowering to you.

It might be something you consider kink, which Stefani Goerlich (2023) defines as "anything that falls outside of the sexual, erotic, or relational norm." It might be a fetish, which she defines as "sexual attraction to an object or body part that is not usually seen as sexual." As an example, a relatively common fetish is feet, which means feet are sexy to you and you are aroused by them. You might be interested, or have secretly wondered if you are interested, in BDSM. BDSM stands for bondage, dominance, sadism, and masochism. According to Dr. Goerlich (2023), this is an umbrella term that includes "an exchange of *control*" (bondage and domination), "an exchange of *authority*" (dominance and submission), or focusing on "giving and receiving *sensation*" (sadism and masochism). While it may seem taboo, about 86% of Americans have either tried BDSM or are interested in doing so (Bedbible Research Center, 2024), so it's probably not as "weird" as you think it is. And it's also ok if it is outside the "norms" and not very many people are interested in what you're interested in. Each of us is unique. If you want more information about kink, fetishes, or BDSM, I highly recommend *With Sprinkles on Top* by Stefani Goerlich (2023).

Emotions related to sexuality don't just apply to desires or preferences. Sometimes the aspects of our sexuality that we need to explore include gender identity, gender expression, sexual orientation, or relational orientation. Understanding who you are is a critical part of being able to love who you are. Gender identity refers to your internal sense of your gender, or how you feel. Gender expression is the outward expression of your gender. This can include pronouns, clothing, and mannerisms. If you want to explore more about this, I recommend *You and Your Gender Identity* by Dara Hoffman-Fox (2017). Sexual orientation is who you are attracted to, emotionally, romantically, and/or physically. It also relates to which element is most important to you. Is emotional attraction most important? Or is romantic attraction or physical attraction primary for you? Relational orientation refers to how you structure relationships and express commitment. Regarding relational orientation, communication and consent are vital. Changing the structure of your relationship doesn't change patterns of deception or other violations of the relational contract. If you need more information about relational orientations other than monogamy, *Polysecure* by Jessica Fern (2020) or *The Ethical Slut* by Janet Hardy and Dossie Easton (2017) might be helpful.

The third question shifts to focusing on the external influences that shaped your beliefs about sex and relationships. "How did my upbringing, past relationships, or cultural background shape my emotional connection to sexuality?" This explores the messages, role models, and experiences that influenced your emotional framework around sexuality. This is a broader perspective that considers where your emotional beliefs come from. As you explore this question, consider the family you grew up in, the cultures you are or were part of, your religious background and beliefs, your experience in current and past relationships, and your understanding of societal expectations. What did you learn about your permission to understand and express yourself? What parts of that do you want to take with you and which parts do you want to leave behind?

Emotional safety is the foundation of sexual fulfillment. If you don't feel emotionally safe, it is difficult to fully experience pleasure, vulnerability, or deep connection. This ties back to the Hierarchy of Needs we discussed throughout this book and focused on in Chapter 6. We have to fill the bottom levels of the pyramid to reach the top ones. This applies to sexuality as well. It also applies within relationships. It is never ok to make someone do something they don't feel safe with. Connection does not include coercion, manipulation, or deception. If you are feeling coerced, manipulated, or if deception is part of your current relationship, set the boundaries you need to keep yourself safe. If you feel as though the only way you'll get your needs met is through coercion, manipulation, or deception, you will not be able to build long-term peace, connection, or joy with those as part of the equation. Stop any behaviors in those categories and process through why you turned to those as you tried to advocate for yourself.

It's important to honor yourself and anyone you're connected to throughout this process. As we've discussed throughout this book, consent is vital. Communication is essential. As you explore these topics, stay aligned with who you are and who you want to be. Factor in empathy and compassion for yourself and for others. Clearly communicate any changes in boundaries. Use the tools we've talked about to work through internal struggles that come up and any differences within your relationship. Talk with your therapist, either your individual therapist or your relational therapist or both, if needed as you work to understand who you are individually and relationally.

Exercise 14–2:

1. What emotions arise when you think about your sexuality?
2. Have you been taught or learned that certain emotions around sex are "bad" or "wrong"? If so, how has that impacted you in the past? How is it currently impacting you?
3. How did your upbringing, past relationships, or cultural background shape your emotional connection to sexuality?

Physical Exploration

Physical exploration of sexuality is a deeply personal and highly individualized process that should be approached with intentionality. Consent is vital. Consent isn't just about others; it's also about yourself. Don't force yourself to do something you aren't comfortable with. Often the journey of sexual self-discovery is intertwined with past experiences, cultural messaging, and personal beliefs. This is why we explore the emotional aspect first – so that physical exploration comes from a place of safety, self-compassion, and genuine curiosity rather than obligation, pressure, or unresolved trauma.

As we've discussed, societal norms, religious teachings, or past experiences can create internalized shame, fear, or discomfort regarding our body and sexuality. By addressing emotions first, we can approach physical exploration with openness rather than apprehension. This reduces the likelihood of triggers, distress, and reinforcement of dysfunctional patterns. Although I've stated this multiple times, I want to reiterate that you get to decide when and how to take these steps. You don't have to do anything you aren't ready to do.

The first question related to this aspect of healing is "What structure is needed for you to be able to take this step?" As you consider this question, approach it with curiosity rather than judgment, incorporating self-empathy and self-compassion. Do you feel safest exploring this by yourself? Or within your relationship? Interpersonal transparency is understanding how much of ourselves we feel safe sharing with others. What level do you feel comfortable sharing about this within your relationship?

If this topic is best explored within your relationship, what boundaries do you need around being touched? Factor your relational contract into the equation. If your relational contract includes boundaries around communication related to physical exploration of yourself, honor those boundaries. If those boundaries prevent you from being able to take these steps, review the boundaries, consider why they were set up and if there might be additional ways to ensure emotional safety, and communicate within your relationship before taking any steps to change them. If you need help navigating this, talk to your relational or individual therapist.

Once you've set up the structure that feels safest for you, honoring your needs and the commitments you've made to self and others, we can move toward physical exploration. Physical exploration of sexuality is not about forced masturbation or having more sex. It can include masturbation or sex if you want it to, but it doesn't need to include either. Don't include either until you feel interested in them and ready to take those steps. Physical exploration is about creating a safe, non-judgmental connection with your own body at a level that is comfortable for you. You're getting to know yourself and what you like and don't like.

A good starting point is learning how your body feels and responds to different sensations. In Chapter 13 we talked about redefining the word "sensual" as relating to connecting to ourselves through experiencing our senses. Explore how your body responds to different touch, temperature, or movement. Notice where tension or relaxation shows up and consider how that relates to your emotions.

You can include sexual experiences as part of these steps, but you don't have to. Whether or not you include sexual experiences, make sure to include non-sexual ones as well. For example, pay attention to the temperature of the water in the shower, to the texture of the sheets or blankets on your bed or on a couch or chair. Feel the warmth of the sun on your skin when you're outside or by a window. Feel the wind as it blows across your face or arms. Feel the ground beneath your feet as you walk. Feel the muscles in your body as you stretch or exercise. Pay attention to how your body responds when you take a deep breath or let your breath out. Consider what pleasure and comfort feel like in non-sexual ways.

These steps help to reframe self-touch as connection to yourself. They encourage embodiment, which is feeling fully present in your body rather than detached or critical of it. Let these steps unfold in a way that fits you, aligns with your beliefs and values, and the commitments you've made to yourself and others. Don't feel forced or pressured. Observe yourself and learn about your body's responses. Recognize that everyone's body and physical responses are different. The goal isn't to fit into a prescribed idea of sexuality, but to discover what is authentic and connecting for you. This process is about developing a respectful, trusting, and intuitive relationship with your own body.

Exercise 14–3:

1. What structure is needed for you to be able to take this step? How does that align with your boundaries for yourself and your relational contract if you are in a relationship?
2. Over the next several days or weeks, what steps can you take to learn what your body feels? How will you keep track of what you learn?

Arousal Exploration

As we mentioned earlier, exploring the arousal domain bridges emotional and physical domains, helping you to understand what you want and how you want it. Currently, the word arousal is almost always used in relation to sexual responses, but the basic definition of the word is to awaken or evoke a strong feeling (Collins English Dictionary, n.d.). In this case, we are focusing on awakening the feeling of wanting to connect with your sexuality, whatever that means for you. As with other aspects we've discussed, this is about curiosity and self-awareness, and connection, not about any specific goal or expectation.

Arousal is more than just a physical response. It often includes a physical response, but not always. Remember our discussion around arousal non-concordance in Chapter 12? Sometimes we feel arousal, but our bodies don't respond physically. Arousal is a complex interplay of emotions, thoughts, sensory experiences, and physiological responses. It's influenced by factors such as emotional safety, trust, connection, cultural background, religious beliefs or conditioning, and personal narratives.

Arousal is highly individual. It's not just about desire. It's also about the conditions that allow it to develop and thrive. Exploring arousal means gaining a deeper understanding of what excites you, makes you feel safe, and helps you connect with yourself and possibly others. It's about discovering who you are rather than producing responses you think you should have. It's not a performance or a requirement. It also changes over time and varies depending on multiple factors.

Rosemary Basson (2000) introduced the idea that there are two types of arousal, spontaneous and responsive. Spontaneous arousal happens suddenly and without an external cause. Responsive arousal is in reaction to a situation, sensation, emotional state, or connection. Neither one is better than the other. Recognizing that both exist can help you to better understand yourself.

Arousal can be activated by internal or external stimuli. Internal stimuli might include thoughts, emotions, or fantasies. External stimuli might include sensory experiences, touch, or relational dynamics. As we talked about in Chapter 11, we have both an accelerator and brakes. This section focuses primarily on what pushes on your accelerator. Previous chapters have helped process through what pushes on your brakes. Be aware of what you've learned about yourself from previous chapters and honor yourself if any of this material pushes on your brakes. Give yourself time and space to listen to the messages you're receiving from yourself and determine the steps and timing that are best for you.

Exercise 14–4:

1. What types of thoughts, memories, or fantasies are arousing to you?
2. Thinking back on the work you did in the previous section, what types of touch or sensory experiences increase your connection to your body and feel pleasurable?
3. How is your arousal impacted by your emotional state? Do you find arousal easier in certain moods? What makes you feel safest?
4. What disconnects you from arousal? How do you know when you become disconnect from it?
5. Are there any cultural, societal, or religious messages that influence how you experience or suppress arousal?

Super Short Summary:

Seeing yourself and understanding yourself is the first step toward rebuilding your sexual world in a way that brings you joy and connection. Self-exploration is not about "fixing" yourself. It's about creating an empowered relationship with your body, your emotions, and your authentic self. Self-exploration includes three domains: emotional, physical, and arousal. Physical is connection to your body. Emotional is connection to your heart. Arousal connects physical and emotional, focusing on understanding what feels safe for you, what excites you, and what aligns with your values and sense of self.

Chapter Questions:

1. What did you connect to the most in this chapter?
2. What steps are you taking to apply this material to your life?

15

Connection

Sexual Connection

The connection component of late recovery focuses on sexual connection. Sexual connection is deeply intertwined with emotional safety. In this final chapter on healing sexuality, we'll integrate all we've learned throughout this book and specifically what we've discussed in the last four chapters to help you create a fulfilling, congruent, and meaningful connection with yourself and within your relationship if you are in one.

Like any type of connection, sexual connection starts with emotional safety. One of the most powerful conversations I've been part of around emotional safety related to sex was in one of the classes I took as part of my PhD program. The class was called *Trauma, Drama, and Kink* and it was taught by Jasmine Johnson and King Noire (Johnson & Noire, 2021). There were about 90 of us in the online class and they asked us to type in the chat what we thought made sex emotionally safe. The answers boiled down to a few general categories, which seemed to apply universally as those of us attending the class were from various educational, cultural, and religious backgrounds, across different genders, sexual orientations, and relational orientations. According to that conversation, sexual connection is emotionally safe when each person is seen, respected, and their vulnerability is honored, interactions are balanced, there are limits and boundaries, and trust has been built. Additionally, interactive communication is essential, as is lack of judgment, although lack of judgment **does not** mean automatic compliance.

Emotional safety is not just a personal experience. It is reinforced through structure and boundaries, although structure and boundaries are highly individual and will differ for each person and each relationship and will likely change and develop over time. Emotional safety is built on trust. As we mentioned in Chapter 3, trust is behavior over time. Trust develops when emotional safety is consistently honored. This applies to both ourselves and our relationships. Trust in ourselves comes from patterns of identifying and honoring internal emotional, physical, and relational signals. Relational trust develops from ongoing patterns of behavior over time that includes consent, communication, and concern.

As with other levels of connection to self and others, healthy sexual connection is not about incongruent or forced performance. It's about being fully present, identify, communicating, and honoring needs, limits, and desires. Boundaries are essential to maintaining safety throughout the process and maximizing connection.

DOI: 10.4324/9781003623359-19

Boundaries Around Sexual Connection

Previous chapters have provided information and tools to help you connect to yourself, understand your emotional responses, and learn how your body responds, what it likes and what it dislikes. The Restarting Sexual Connection worksheet, available at ConnectedRecoveryTraining.com, can help walk you through combining that material into a structure for sexual connection. This exercise can be done individually or relationally.

It starts with defining different levels of sexual connection. This may be connection that includes only yourself. It may be connection that includes only interactions with others. It could be both. Use it in a way that fits best for you. This worksheet includes levels 0–5. If you prefer to use a different scale, create one that works for you. Maybe you prefer 0–10, or you prefer colors. You get to decide how best to define this. I recommend using a structure that allows you to move items around as you will likely make changes as you create this. You might create a virtual document that lets you cut and paste items, or a whiteboard that allows you to erase them. Maybe you use pieces of paper you can move around as you sort through how to make sense of the different levels.

One client I had, who gave me permission to share this, used a magnetic whiteboard. She chose to use 0–10 and divided the board in half vertically because she included both emotional and physical aspects of each level. She wrote each element on a small magnetic strip, so she could move them around on the board as she sorted through how best to organize them based on her individual experience and beliefs. In her case, she used this to determine how to move forward with a new relationship and it helped her to ensure that she developed trust and connection as that relationship developed. This connected these steps to the concept of relational currency that we talked about in Chapter 9.

If you are using this exercise within a relationship, I recommend you agree on a general format for the scale (0–5, or 0–10, or colors, or something else), then define the levels individually first. Be as specific as possible. It's absolutely ok to decide there are certain things that you are never ok with, or at the very least, are not currently ok with.

Once you've defined them individually, if you are in a relationship, figure out the best way to share them with each other and work toward developing a scale both of you understand. Sometimes this can be a difficult step to take if you've felt shame around sexual connection or if you've experienced trauma related to it, whether in your current relationship or in other situations. It can also sometimes be difficult to have this conversation if there was coercion, manipulation, abuse, deception, or betrayal in the relationship. It's ok to need help to have this conversation. Work with your relational and/or individual therapist to get any support you need.

Once you've created levels that fit for you, and for your relationship if you're using this tool within a relationship, you can use those levels to communicate about what you're comfortable with at any given time. If you are at different levels, connection maxes out at the highest level each person in the relationship is comfortable with. For example, if one person is ok with level five interactions, and another is ok with up to level three interactions, all connection would be at level three or below.

This maximizes your connection because it allows you to clearly define boundaries. As we've talked about throughout this book, boundaries provide the safety and freedom to connect at the level that is best for us. This tool specifically addresses the "domino effect" in sexual connection. The domino effect is the idea that once one step has been taken, the next steps are inevitable. It removes our ability to pause, reassess, or stop sexual connection, removing agency and autonomy from the process. This can happen externally or internally.

The external domino effect refers to pressure to continue. For example, if you start kissing, it has to lead to sex. This can be due to cultural conditioning, coercion, or manipulation. It's founded on the false belief that participating in sexual activity creates a situation where someone "owes" continued participation. There are many commonly used phrases that relate to this. "But you started it..." "You got me all worked up. Don't leave me hanging." "You can't tease me like this." "I thought you wanted this." "You knew what you were doing when we started this." These phrases can also include threats like "If you won't, I'll find someone who will."

Sometimes the domino effect can be internal. The internal domino effect happens when we feel unable to stop once we start. Not because someone is pressuring us, but because we don't know how or when to stop. We struggle to recognize our own emotions, needs, and boundaries in real time. This can happen when our boundaries aren't clearly defined within ourselves. It can also happen when we don't trust our own experience or don't know how to give ourselves time and space to pause and process when needed. It can be due to fear of disappointing someone or disrupting the moment. It can also be due to trauma responses, which we talked about in Chapter 1.

Sexual interactions aren't like getting on a waterslide, where once you push off, you can't stop or turn around. You don't have to keep going if you start. You can stop whenever you want to or need to. You can pause whenever you want to or need to. It's crucial to set up a structure where you're able to stop or pause, so you can feel safe, which allows you to connect with yourself and others without being afraid that it will automatically lead to something you're not ready for or worrying how to say no if things escalate.

One of the biggest barriers to reconnecting sexually, especially after betrayal, trauma, or other major relational struggles, is fear of losing control over the process. Many people avoid intimacy completely because they don't trust that they or those they are connected to will stop if needed or that boundaries will be honored. Defining levels and communicating about each person's current comfort level helps allow each to feel comfortable exploring because it removes the pressure to go beyond what they are comfortable with. It's important to recognize that stating the level you're at does not mean you have to do anything. It's about possibilities, not obligations. For example, if kissing is on one of the levels you're ok with, it doesn't mean you have to kiss. It means you're ok with them asking "Can I give you a kiss?" or possibly instigating a kiss, depending on how you'd prefer to be communicated with.

Another critical element of this tool is recognizing that trust is built by honoring boundaries, not by testing or pushing against them. It's important that each person respects and protects the boundaries that are set and communicated. Don't push someone else to go further than what they've said they are comfortable with. When each partner feels safe, sexual interactions have the potential to become genuinely connecting.

The questions on the Restarting Sexual Connection worksheet help to set up additional boundaries to help you as you navigate through communicating changes related to the levels of sexual connection. The first question considers how you might instigate connection. Are each of you ok with non-verbal initiation, meaning can interactions at the level you're comfortable with be started without a verbal request? Or would you prefer them to ask you if you're ok with it first? As a sidenote, if you're not sure, default to asking. "Can I give you a hug?" or "Would you be ok with a kiss?"

The second question considers how you might recognize you aren't interested when a request for connection is made and how to potentially communicate that to yourself or within your relationship. Requests for connection, whether physical, emotional, or sexual, are inherently vulnerable. Rejection can feel painful, triggering insecurity or reinforcing existing wounds, especially if those in the relationship have experienced trauma or disconnection. The person who isn't interested may feel guilt, confusion, or be afraid of hurting the person who made the request. This can lead to avoidance or compliance rather than genuine connection. Proactively discussing how to respond helps to foster connection. This allows each individual to consider what they might need from the situation and provides the opportunity to incorporate empathy into future interactions at deeper levels.

The third helps plan for how you might pause or stop the connection if you get triggered or if you need a break. This reinforces safety, making it easier to engage. It helps to prevent shutting down or dissociating by giving you specific steps and words to use that maximize your ability to connect with your needs, allowing you to stay present. It increases each person's ability to understand and honor when an interaction is paused or stopped and normalizes flexibility and communication.

Exercise 15–1:

1. Using the Restarting Sexual Connection worksheet, what structure would you like to use to define levels of sexual connection? Use that structure to define what different levels look like for you. If you are in a relationship, figure out the best steps to share those and determine steps that fits for each of you.
2. How would you like physical and sexual connection to be instigated?
3. What would you like incorporated into communicating that someone isn't interested in connection when a request is made?
4. What phrases could be used to stop or pause sexual connection?

The fourth question on the worksheet focuses on identifying and potentially sharing specific desires or preferences that might make sexual experiences fulfilling for you. This step emphasizes communication and consent, but it's essential to recognize the level of vulnerability involved and factor that into the equation, especially if past experiences have caused unwanted pain, disconnection, or trauma.

Understanding your own desires is the first step in this part of the process. We've walked through understanding yourself at different levels throughout this book, helping you to know who you are and what you like and dislike. As we mentioned at the beginning of Chapter 14, starting in the introduction, we considered what you like and don't like. The work you did in Chapter 14 helped to apply the tools and insights you've developed throughout this process to physical connection and then considered your arousal template. Take some time to dig deeper into that topic and consider your sexual desires.

Exercise 15–2:

1. What specific activities, types of touch, emotional connection, and environments are you interested in?
2. What helps you feel safe and connected? What does clear communication look like for you, including verbal interactions and non-verbal cues? What kinds of touch, words, or actions help you feel cared for and desired?
3. What are you interested in exploring? Are there any new ideas or practices that are intriguing to you?

Communicating the answers to the questions above can help maximize the connection in interpersonal interactions. This may not be a step you're ready to take, especially if you've previously shared desires before in this relationship, or in a previous relationship, and the experience caused disconnection or trauma. For example, if you shared something you wanted or liked and you felt you were shamed for it, or it was used as a weapon against you. Or if you asked for something and the request was repeatedly ignored. Sharing your desires can feel deeply vulnerable. You don't have to share everything at once or at all.

Identify and process the emotions that come up for you as you consider what you want to share and how you want to share it. Process through those emotions to determine what steps might be helpful to repair connection in that area, or what boundaries you need moving forward. Use the tools we've talked about throughout this book to determine if and how you want to share anything you process. Due to the vulnerability related to this topic, carefully choose the time and place to share and take the steps to get support in the ways that are best for you. Stay in your hula hoop and express your emotions, needs, and experiences. Incorporate empathy and compassion for yourself and for those you're sharing with. Honor your boundaries and theirs.

If you choose to share any part of your list of what you're interested in sexually, recognize that if one person lists something that another isn't comfortable with, it doesn't mean they have to do it. Consent is vital. Each person has the right to say "yes, we can try that," or "no, I'm not comfortable with that," or "I can't do that, but could we try this?" You can also apply those three levels of consent to interactions with yourself. Consider different sexual experiences. Some you might be interested in. Others you might not be. Some might spark some interest, but only in a specific way or with specific boundaries. Whether your connection is individual or relational, you don't have to do anything. Respect the boundaries of each person involved, including yourself.

The final question considers what you might want or need after sexual connection to ensure the connection you felt is maximized. This can be a critical part of rebuilding sexual connection. For many people, especially those with a history of traumatic experiences related to sexual connection, what happens immediately after sexual connection can help shape whether the experience is positive and bonding or disconnecting and dysregulating. Each person has unique needs. As with each part of the process, identifying, communicating, and honoring those needs helps to maximize connection. Some people need additional physical closeness. Others need emotional reassurance. Some need space or self-reflection. Understanding each person's needs helps to prevent misunderstandings and ensure that each person feels safe and valued. As with other types of boundaries, honoring these boundaries strengthens trust and builds safety.

Exercise 15–3:

1. What might make sexual connection best for you?
2. How much of this do you feel comfortable sharing? Explore any fears or concerns around sharing this within a relationship.
3. What do you need or want following sexual connection?

Defining Sexual Success

Sexual success isn't about achieving specific physical outcomes, although it can be difficult to make that shift mentally. The goal of sexual interaction is to connect with yourself, and to connect within your relationship if you are including relational interactions. In order to understand sexual success, we need to redefine what "sex" means for you. Common definitions focus on specific acts, such as penetration (oral, vaginal, or anal), and bodily responses, such as orgasm or ejaculation. These elements may sometimes, or even often, be part of a successful sexual experience for you, but they don't define success.

Sexual success has five elements, which relate directly to the work we've done throughout this book. They are:

1. Building and/or strengthening connection to yourself and within your relationship.
2. Ensuring that each person has bodily autonomy, which means control over your own body and what you choose to do with it.
3. Identifying and communicating boundaries and needs throughout the process.
4. Staying congruent with yourself and giving others the space to stay congruent with themselves.
5. Maintaining emotional safety throughout the process.

Let's explore these in more detail.

Sexual success begins with connection to self. This starts with identifying, understanding, and honoring your own needs, emotions, and wants. This involves tuning into your body and emotions, listening to yourself, and believing yourself. In the last chapter, we considered emotional attunement to self and physical attunement to self. In Chapter 11, we talked about understanding what sexy means to you. In Chapter 12 we discussed sexual trauma and abuse and the impact traumatic experiences may have had on you. In Chapter 13 we walked through reclaiming and redefining elements related to your sexuality. In Chapter 14, we began the process of exploring how your body and mind responds and what it likes and doesn't like. Taking this to the next level, this section focuses specifically on what you like sexually.

As we work toward redefining sexual success, recognize that the focus is pleasure, joy, and connection with self and potentially with your relationship. As Emily Nagoski says, "pleasure is the measure" (2021). The word "pleasure" often has a sexual, or even shameful, connotation in today's society, ranging back over at least 80 years, as the island in the 1940s Disney animated film *Pinocchio* includes "Pleasure Island," an amusement park full of gambling and smoking cigars and gluttony (Disney, Sharpsteen, & Luske, 1940). This highlights the depth of societal shame founded in puritanical beliefs that enjoyment is sinful. Merriam-Webster (n.d.-b) defines pleasure as "a source of delight or joy." Joy is "loving what's true" (Nagoski, 2016).

Combining these into one definition, pleasure is something that helps you to love who you are and love what you're experiencing. The first element of sexual success is that the experience helps you understand yourself better, connect more deeply with yourself, and love who you are and what is true for you. If this connection includes a partner or partners, it helps each person to connect with themselves, honor and love who they are, and it helps each to connect interpersonally in that way that fits best for them.

Autonomy is essential. Autonomy means having control over your own body and your own choices. As we talked about earlier in this chapter, emotionally safe sex identifies and respects boundaries and limits for each person. Even in situations where control or authority is part of the desired structure, such as when BDSM or kink is part of the dynamic, it's about "an exchange" (Goerlich, 2023) and each person has the ability to stop or pause at any point in the process. Incorporation of consent is necessary for any situation to be empowering and connecting. Sexual success through the lens of autonomy means that each person felt empowered to say "yes" or "no" at any point without fear of judgment or rejection, each person felt respected and supported, and each experienced the interaction as a collaborative process rather than a one-sided expectation.

The third element, relating to the communication of boundaries and needs throughout the experience, first requires that each person has the tools and opportunity to identify their needs, and being able to communicate them and feeling heard and respected around them. This is often a very vulnerable step. It's more damaging to have our needs not met if we overtly identify and ask for them. If we know what we really want and we know we've communicated it, it's more difficult when it's not incorporated into the situation. Figure out the level of communication that is best for you, as we talked about earlier in this chapter when discussing the Restarting Sexual Connection worksheet.

Staying congruent with yourself throughout the process is critical. You've done the work throughout this book to better understand who you are and who you want to be, behaviorally, internally, and relationally. Sexual success includes aligning yourself with your core values, emotions, and comfort levels. It's about being honest with yourself and not acting out of guilt, shame, fear, or obligation. It means honoring your internal "yes" or "no" and not compromising yourself to meet internal or external expectations. It means staying true to yourself throughout the experience.

Emotional safety is foundational for sexual success. An emotionally safe environment makes each individual feel supported and respected and allows for open communication. It also factors in an awareness of and empathy for past experiences and the impact of those experiences on each individual and possibly on the relational dynamics. This includes recognizing potential triggers and incorporating a structure that allows interactions to be stopped or paused at any point in the process without fear, helping each person to feel emotionally secure and be less guarded.

Sexual success is not about achieving specific outcomes, it's about the quality of the experience. The work we've done to better understand ourselves and the experiences we've gone through, reclaiming and redefining different aspects of our experiences, and more deeply connecting to ourselves through self-exploration, culminate in the ability to create experiences where you feel safe, respected, and authentic. Where you can feel confident because you know what's true, and experience joy, because you love what's true (Nagoski, 2016).

Exercise 15–4:

1. How would you define sexual success?
2. What does pleasure mean to you and how does this align or misalign with your understanding of how society and the cultures you are part of define it?
3. What steps might be helpful to recognize and honor your own needs, emotions, and boundaries in sexual experiences?
4. What steps might help ensure that your sexual experiences align with your core values and your authentic self?
5. What boundaries might be needed to make sexual connection safe for you and how can you communicate those boundaries?

Super Short Summary:

Sexual connection starts with emotional safety. Healthy sexual connection is about being fully present, identifying, communicating, and honoring needs, limits, and desires. Sexual success isn't about achieving specific physical outcomes, it's about learning to connect with yourself, and to connect within your relationship, if you are including relational interactions, where you are safe, respected, and able to be authentically you. It's about loving who you are.

Chapter Questions:

---

1. What did you connect to the most in this chapter?
2. What steps are you taking to apply this material to your life?

Conclusion

You've made it!! We've covered each of the five components as they relate to early, middle, and late recovery.

Healing from betrayal, infidelity, and problematic sexual behaviors is a journey. It requires courage, a willingness to explore the truth, and deep personal and relational work. Recognize that recovery is not linear. It is an ongoing process of repair, reconnection, and restoration that takes time, patience, and a willingness to engage in both self-exploration and relational healing. The work we've done has helped to build a foundation of emotional safety, deepen connection with ourselves and others, and heal sexuality. I encourage you to continue the work we've started, making this process your own and applying the concepts and tools in the way that works best for you. Review the material and tools as needed. If you are a parent and are concerned about how to address issues related to parenting following betrayal and breaking generational patterns, there is a separate chapter following this conclusion addressing both of those topics.

Healing is possible. Peace is possible. Whether your process focuses on individual recovery or includes both individual and relational recovery, you can feel whole again. You are more than your past, more than your pain. It is possible to build a life that is whole, connected, and fulfilling.

As you walk this path, remember, you don't have to do this alone. Your support systems can provide the encouragement and accountability needed to sustain change. By facing the truth, embracing healing and building connection with yourself and others, you can create a life you love. Healing is not just about recovering from the past. It's about building a future.

This isn't the end. It's the beginning.

Special Topic

16

Parenting Following Betrayal and Breaking Generational Patterns

While not everyone dealing with betrayal has children, parenting in the wake of betrayal, infidelity, or problematic sexual behavioral patterns presents unique challenges. This chapter focuses on those challenges and on changing intergenerational patterns. I use the word "children" throughout this chapter. This applies to children regardless of age, from toddlers to adults.

What to Share and How to Share It

Every situation is different, so what's best will differ for each family. What you choose to disclose and how to disclose it needs to be thoughtfully considered. It is crucial to find a balance between honesty and protecting your children, no matter how old they are, from unnecessary pain. Once information is shared, it cannot be reversed, but not sharing information at some level often makes the situation much worse.

Children, regardless of age, are perceptive. Even when nothing is overtly shared and each parent does everything they can to hide the pain they are dealing with, they often sense tension, emotional distress, or changes in family dynamics. Denying that something is wrong when they can clearly sense that something major is happening creates confusion and feels like a form of gaslighting. Pretending everything is fine can make children question their own realities and instincts.

The most basic level of communication around betrayal is claiming responsibility around the pain caused. Often the parent who has been betrayed has more overt emotional responses, which can lead children to incorrectly assume that the parent who has been betrayed is responsible for the situation. It's important for the parent who has betrayed to convey that they did something that caused significant pain to the other parent, whether or not you decide any details should be shared. This provides context for the emotions that children may sense and is an important step toward amends.

Whatever level of sharing ends up being right for you and your family, avoid triangulation. Children should never be put in a position where they feel they have to choose between their parents. Don't use them as emotional support or confidantes. This places an unfair burden on them. Do the work to be able to listen to your children's emotions or concerns without putting them in a position where they need to provide you with support. Don't deny your emotions because that is similar to gaslighting. Do the work so you

DOI: 10.4324/9781003623359-21

have tools and a support system that provides you with the ability to process through your emotions without involving your children in the equation. Your children deserve the freedom to maintain relationships with their parents without being placed in the middle of the conflict.

In some cases, children become aware of betrayal by directly discovering evidence of the behaviors, overhearing conversations, or noticing significant changes in their home environment. In other cases, they may just sense that something is wrong. If they are aware of the betrayal, they may feel trapped by that knowledge, believing that either way, they are betraying one parent. If they talk about what they know, they may feel they are betraying the parent who committed the problematic behaviors. If they stay silent, they may feel like they are betraying the parent who has been betrayed. It's essential to let them know that it's not their responsibility to create safety or protect either parent. Give them a safe space to process through their emotions.

I highly recommend each child has their own individual therapist if at all possible. I also recommend that they are given space to process in those sessions without the parents requiring that they or their clinician disclose what is discussed in their therapy sessions, even if they are under 18 and the parents can legally require the information to be shared. They need a neutral space where they don't have to filter, and they can explore what they're going through in a healthy and constructive way. That doesn't mean that parents should ignore their instincts if they feel the clinician is making the situation worse rather than helping. As we discussed in the introduction, holding a mental health license does not mean every clinician will be a good fit. Outside of concerns such as those, I recommend not micromanaging your child's therapeutic support process.

Whenever possible, it is important for both parents to be on the same page around what they want to share with their children. This helps to minimize confusion and triangulation, reduce anxiety, and provides a more stable foundation for their emotional processing. As important as this is, it should not come at the expense of pretending the situation is different from what it is or placing blame on the person who has been betrayed.

The best approach is for parents to work together, if at all possible, to provide an age-appropriate, truthful narrative that does not villainize or excuse behavior, but focuses on healing and moving forward. This doesn't mean lying about what happened. If there's information you don't feel is appropriate to share, state that you don't think that would be helpful to talk about rather than lying about it. Try not to contradict each other as this places children in a position where they are pressured to take sides and decide which parent to believe. Strive for clarity, honesty, and a united front that prioritizes their well-being above all else.

Work to prevent your children from feeling like they must choose between their parents. If your relationship ends, recognize that while you may be losing your partner, they are still your children's parent. Honor their relationship with their other parent, even in difficult circumstances. Do not use them as pawns or attempt to poison their perception of their other parent.

Parenting in the aftermath of betrayal requires balance – being honest without oversharing, creating an emotional space for children without making them responsible for your emotions, and protecting them without hiding the truth. This is difficult even in the best situations. Navigating it while dealing with the aftermath of betrayal in your relationship is often incredibly overwhelming. Recognize that you will make mistakes along the way. Make sure you have support to help you when you make mistakes, so your children are not responsible for taking care of you when that happens.

If safety concerns are present, seek additional professional help to ensure the well-being of your children. Referring to the Hierarchy of Needs, safety is most important. In most cases, this is not part of the equation, so the focus is on fostering an environment where your children feel secure, heard, loved, and supported as they navigate through this chapter.

Exercise Special Topic–1:

1. What do you think your children know about the situation?
2. How much do you think would be helpful for each of them to know? Factor in their age and what you know about the way they process emotions.
3. What does your significant other(s) think would be helpful for each child to know? If there is a significant difference between this answer and the answer above, seek professional guidance as you work to find a balance.
4. What information have you as a team decided will be shared with each of your children? How will you address any additional questions they have?
5. What type of support does each of your children have? What additional support might be helpful?
6. What support do you need so you can provide support to your children? How will you address mistakes you make in this aspect of the recovery process?

Supporting Your Children's Emotional Needs

Again, I highly recommend you provide your children with therapeutic support. They need a neutral place to process through their experience. Beyond providing therapeutic support, recognize that there are other ways your children may be impacted by the recovery process.

The overwhelming nature of betrayal can sometimes lead parents to unintentionally neglect their children's emotional needs. This is understandable as the recovery process takes so much energy, effort, and time, similar to a situation where a family member is dealing with a significant medical issue. There's only so much each of us has to give. If you're aware of this, you can take steps to work to incorporate additional support to help rebalance this equation. Consider your support system and who might be able to help you by providing your children with extra support.

There are three general ways children deal with familial changes such as those that happen as their parents are going through the recovery process. One is that they become silent, sensing the emotional weight their parents are carrying. They may fear their emotions are too much and they will be a burden. Another potential response, which is founded in similar fears, is working to become perfect or overachieve. This may be due to a desire to make their parents happier, or it may be striving for control in an environment that feels unstable. The third type of response is behavioral struggles, perhaps because they don't know how to handle the pain they're feeling, or in an attempt to get a connection even if it's painful. It may also be that the added emotional weight makes all their emotions feel bigger. Whatever their response, do the work so you're aware of their needs and you can help them get help to process through their emotions and get their needs met.

If the betrayal becomes public, be mindful of the potential social ramifications for your children. They may face questions from their friends, family members, or others. There may be shifts in their friendships. They may struggle with shame or embarrassment. Build a space where they can voice what their experience is and get support to process through it.

Whether or not the betrayal becomes public, it can be confusing for a child to know what is ok to share with others. We talked earlier about how isolating betrayal can be for those who have been betrayed and for those struggling with problematic sexual behaviors. It is also isolating for children. They may feel like they are betraying their parents by discussing what they're going through. They may not know the boundaries around who they can talk to about it, especially in relation to sharing with extended family members or friends. Proactively encourage conversation with you about these topics. Start by asking what their thoughts are and who they would like to include on their support team. Ask what they would like to be able to share with others and what type of support they need around that. With empathy and compassion, share any boundaries you have related to how you would prefer the information to be shared and if there is anyone you would prefer them not to share it with. Make sure they have the support they need, and you aren't creating a "secret basement," as we talked about in Chapter 7. There's a difference between boundaried sharing and silencing someone. Work to ensure that you are fostering an environment that encourages boundaried sharing rather than keeping secrets.

Betrayal can be incredibly consuming. It can take over every aspect of life, making it easy to lose sight of any sense of normalcy. Each of us needs stability. Whenever possible, work to prioritize maintaining routines. Take time to engage in activities that allow space for joy and connection.

Remember that betrayal impacts not only a primary relationship, but the entire family system. And remember you will make mistakes. Awareness of these issues will help you address them.

Exercise Special Topic–2:

1. Who might be able to help provide support for your children through this process?
2. How is each of your children responding to this situation? Which pattern connects to each one of them? What might each specifically need in response to those patterns?
3. Who else knows about the betrayal or the repercussions from it? How might this be impacting your children's social interactions?
4. What boundaries might be helpful around what they share with others? Set up times to communicate with them around those boundaries but listen to them first and factor in what they say and what they need.
5. How can you add structure to their current patterns?
6. What steps can you take to give them and you a break from the pain of this process?

Breaking Generational Patterns

I recognize that this chapter may feel especially heavy to read through. Dealing with our children's pain is often even more challenging than dealing with our own pain or even dealing with our significant other's pain. One of the most common questions I get asked by clients who have children is "how do I change these patterns so my kids never go through the same pain I've gone through?" First of all, the very best thing you can do for your children is to do your own work. Yes, your children have been impacted by the pain you've gone through and the dysfunctional patterns you came into the process with. As you do your work, you model for them how to address the dysfunction. This happens regardless of what you share with them. They see the changes in you and the way you interact with them changes. In developing your own tools, you are helping to show them the tools. As we create healthier approaches, we redefine family rules and interactions, creating a new system that fosters connection rather than fear or shame and allows for healthier communication and healthier connection with self and others. This healthier approach helps to create a family dynamic that is emotionally safe, allows for emotional expression and processing and accountability, building confidence and paving the way to experience joy.

Generational patterns are changed by the same tools you used throughout the recovery process. Bucket-fillers, trauma and escape cycles, containment, processing emotions and needs, processing trauma, advocating for self, and connecting with self and others, all apply to your children as well as you. These tools are founded on principles related to attachment, which apply to everyone. Print the handouts, use the tools, ask your children the questions you ask yourself.

One of the most important aspects of healthy connection to self and others is identifying and processing your emotions and using those emotions to identify your needs, followed by being able to meet those needs in healthy ways. Parents can model and encourage emotional expression by validating their children's emotions, teaching self-regulation skills, and modeling healthy connection by creating a safe environment in which they can share emotions without fear of punishment or rejection. Healthy self-expression can be encouraged through discussing bucket-fillers, having open conversations, and giving them space in which they are accepted for who they are.

Many dysfunctional family patterns come from unresolved trauma responses and patterns related to escape cycles that are modeled and then passed down from one generation to the next. Parents can break these patterns by recognizing their own patterns, such as avoidance of conflict, overcontrolling situations, or shutting down emotions, and consciously choosing emotional awareness and engagement and healthy conflict resolution.

Throughout this book, we've emphasized building support systems and fostering connection. Secure attachment in families is founded on the same building blocks. Encourage self-reflection and self-discovery by creating a system in which it is safe to feel, talk, and connect. Help them to build a strong sense of self through healthy connection with themselves balanced with support from others. Prioritize regular connection, which helps to counteract generational disconnection. Encourage them to define their boundaries and communicate them. Honoring their boundaries teaches them that they should expect others to honor their boundaries and that they are allowed to take steps to protect themselves when their boundaries aren't honored.

Exercise Special Topic–3:

1. What tools from this book might be helpful for your children? How can you start to incorporate those?
2. How are emotions expressed in your home? What do you like about the current patterns and what would you like to change? What steps might be helpful to make those changes?
3. What does communication and connection look like in your home? What do you like about the current patterns and what would you like to change? What steps might be helpful to make those changes?

Many of these changes don't involve big steps. Long-term change is usually gradual. One of the best pieces of advice I ever got as a parent was "if you want them to trust you with the big things, listen to the little ones, because it was always 'big' to them." Listen to your children when they talk to you. Learn who they are. Value what they give you. Make time for them. Put your phone down when you talk to them. Ask them how their day went. I prefer to ask, "what was the best part of your day?" and "what was most difficult for you today?" because I've found those questions produce more specific and connecting responses than "how was your day?" Pay attention to the things that matter to them. Your children sharing those with you are bids for connection. Talk to them about things they are interested in and listen when they talk to you, especially when they are excited about the topic. Tell them you love them. Tell them what you love about them. Encourage them.

Do the work so you can have age-appropriate conversations about intimacy, sex, safety, and bodily autonomy. If those conversations are awkward for you, go talk to your therapist or your friends about those topics until you feel more comfortable with them. Work to identify any shame you have in connection with talking about sex. It's ok to say something like "I know this conversation is awkward. It can be difficult for me to talk about it too." Normalize conversations about sex, relationships, questions about their bodies. It's not about having "the talk" with your kids, it's about making discussions about sex, relationships, and consent a natural part of life. Answer questions with age-appropriate but accurate answers. If you don't know the answer to a question, it's ok to say "I don't know. Let me go figure that out and I'll get back to you." Process through emotions and shame that come up for you, so they don't prevent you from having healthy conversations with your children. Incorporate consent in your interactions with them. I ask my kids' permission before I take photos of them or share those photos with anyone. I ask them if I can hug them or if they want a kiss on the top of their head. Taking this approach helps to ensure they grow up with a healthy, informed, and empowered approach to their bodies, sexuality, and connection with others.

Talk to them about porn. They will be exposed to it. Process through your own emotions and responses first so you can have a conversation that doesn't have added emotional weight from unprocessed emotions. And process through emotions that come up for you in relation to the conversations you have with your kids. The way I approach this with younger children is saying something like, "If you ever come across naked pictures of people, let me know and we can talk about it. Those types of pictures are private." With older kids, I prefer an approach more like "Have you ever come across porn? I know it's pretty common to see it somewhere. Porn is made for entertainment, not education. It doesn't usually show relationships in a healthy way that includes communication, consent, or concern for others. Healthy relationships and interactions include all three of those. Don't use porn for sex ed. It's like using Grand Theft Auto to learn to drive. If you have questions about sex, we can talk about them, or I can connect you with someone else you can talk to if you feel more comfortable with that." Use filtering tools to help protect children from accidental exposure to inappropriate material, but don't rely on them because none of them will work all the time.

Ensure they have accurate information and resources related to medical care and reproductive health. Talk to them about boundaries around sexual activity. If your moral beliefs include beliefs related to sexual interactions, process through your emotions related to those beliefs and work to understand why you believe what you believe, so you can explain it without shaming them. Recognize that they may decide their beliefs align with yours or they may not. Decide what boundaries you need for yourself if their beliefs don't align with yours. Make sure they get accurate and non-shaming sex ed. Don't rely on school health classes to provide accurate and complete information.

The topic of gender identity and expression, sexual orientation, and relational orientation is often a difficult one, but one that is very necessary to navigate through. Societally and culturally, there are enormous amounts of shame and judgment around anything other than alignment with gender assigned at birth and heterosexual monogamous orientation. In the recovery work we outlined, healthy sexuality was saved for the last phase because of the level of vulnerability in it. Gender identity, gender expression, sexual orientation, and relational orientation are some of the most basic and foundational parts of us. Religious beliefs might define how you feel each of these areas can be expressed. You have the right to make those choices for yourself and to determine who you are and how you want to express that. As we just talked about in relation to sexual activity, you children may decide that their beliefs around how to respond to understanding their gender identity, expression, or sexual or relational orientation align with yours or they may not.

Rejecting or judging your child based on any of these is a rejection of them at their deepest core and is incredibly damaging. That doesn't mean you won't have concerns or fears around what they share. Those are normal. We all want our children to be safe and find joy and connection in their lives, and any identities outside of "traditional norms" often produce fear that their life will be more difficult or painful. That fear is likely accurate in many ways. Currently there are significant additional challenges and safety concerns related to any LGBTQ+ identity or orientation. But as I stated earlier, gender identity, gender expression, sexual orientation, and relational orientation are some of the most basic and foundational parts of us, and all identities and orientations are valid. Understanding yourself and your sexuality is essential to healthy connection with self and others. Love and identity are diverse, and that's normal. If your child trusts you enough to tell you about being LGBTQ+, the appropriate response is "Thank you so much for trusting me enough to tell me. I love you so much and you are amazing just the way you are." Reach out and get support for yourself to process through your emotions afterwards but show up for them.

If the last two paragraphs produced strong negative emotions in you, I highly recommend consulting a sex therapist or another clinician with training around rainbow advocacy and processing through the emotions that came up for you. If you don't, you will deeply hurt your children and/or others.

Exercise Special Topic–4:

1. What phrases can you use to start conversations with your children?
2. What do you need to process through to be able to have direct and non-shaming conversations with your children about sex?
3. What do you need to process through so you can connect to your child or children if they share something about their gender identity or expression, sexual orientation, or relational orientation?

Super Short Summary:

You don't need to be perfect. You won't be perfect. You just need to do your own work so you can be present, open, and willing to learn alongside your child. Normalize having open and direct conversations with appropriate boundaries. Teach consent and how to create and enforce healthy boundaries. Teach them to love and honor themselves. Make sure they get accurate, shame-free education. Keep the conversation going throughout their lives. The connection you build with them can be one of the most amazing parts of your life.

Chapter Questions:

1. What did you connect to the most in this chapter?
2. What steps are you taking to apply this material to your life?

References

Ainsworth, M. D. S., Blehar, M. C., Waters, E., & Wall, S. (1978). *Patterns of attachment: A psychological study of the strange situation*. Lawrence Erlbaum Associates.

Alcoholics Anonymous World Services. (2001). *Alcoholics Anonymous: The story of how many thousands of men and women have recovered from alcoholism* (4th ed.). Alcoholics Anonymous World Services.

Allan, R., Edwards, C., & Lee, N. (2022). Cultural adaptations of emotionally focused therapy. *Journal of Couple and Relationship Therapy*, 22(1), 43–63.

American Psychological Association (APA). (2022, November). Intergenerational and historical trauma. *Trauma Psychology News*. https://traumapsychnews.com/2022/11/intergenerational-and-historical-trauma

Bancroft, J., & Janssen, E. (1999). The dual control model of sexual response: A theoretical approach to centrally mediated erectile dysfunction. *Neuroscience & Biobehavioral Reviews*, 24(5), 571–579. https://doi.org/10.1016/S0149-7634(00)00024-5

Barraca, J., & Polanski, T. (2021). Infidelity treatment from an integrative behavioral couple therapy perspective: Explanatory model and intervention strategies. *Journal of Marital and Family Therapy*, 47(4), 909–924.

Bartholomew, K., & Horowitz, L. M. (1991). Attachment styles among young adults: A test of a four-category model. *Journal of Personality and Social Psychology*, 61(2), 226–244. https://doi.org/10.1037/0022-3514.61.2.226

Basson, R. (2000). The female sexual response: A different model. *Journal of Sex & Marital Therapy*, 26(1), 51–65. https://doi.org/10.1080/009262300278641

Bedbible Research Center. (2024, May 15). How common is BDSM [Facts & Statistics]. *Bedbible*. https://bedbible.com/bdsm-statistics-facts-stats

Black, C. (1982). *It will never happen to me: Growing up with addiction as youngsters, adolescents, and adults*. MAC Printing.

Bowen, M. (1978). *Family therapy in clinical practice*. Jason Aronson.

Bowlby, J. (1982). Attachment and loss: Retrospect and Prospect. *American Journal of Orthopsychiatry*, 52(4), 664–678. https://doi.org/10.1111/j.1939-0025.1982.tb01456.x

Bradshaw, J. (1988). *Healing the shame that binds you*. Health Communications.

Brown, B. (2010, June). *The power of vulnerability* [Video]. TED Conferences. www.ted.com/talks/brene_brown_the_power_of_vulnerability

Brown, B. (2012). *Daring greatly: How the courage to be vulnerable transforms the way we live, love, parent, and lead*. Gotham Books.

Cambridge University Press. (n.d.). Consent. *Cambridge dictionary*. https://dictionary.cambridge.org/us/dictionary/english/consent

Carnes, P. (2001). *Facing the shadow: Starting sexual and relationship recovery*. Gentle Path Press.

Caudill, J. (2012). *My personal compass*. [Unpublished Handout].

Caudill, J., & Drake, D. (2020). *Full disclosure: Seeking truth after sexual betrayal. Volume 1: How disclosure can help you heal*. Kintsugi Recovery Partners.

Centers for Disease Control and Prevention (CDC). (2016a). *About the CDC-Kaiser ACE study*. US Department of Health and Human Services. www.cdc.gov/violenceprevention/aces/about.html

Centers for Disease Control and Prevention (CDC). (2016b). *Preventing Adverse Childhood Experiences (ACEs): Leveraging the best available evidence*. US Department of Health and Human Services. www.cdc.gov/violenceprevention/aces/preventingace-datastories.html

Clairmont, P. (1998). *Normal is just a setting on your dryer*. Thomas Nelson.

Collins English Dictionary. (n.d.). Arouse. *Collins dictionary*. www.collinsdictionary.com/us/dictionary/english/arouse

Disney, W. (Producer), & Sharpsteen, B., & Luske, H. (Directors). (1940). Pinocchio [Film]. Walt Disney Productions.

Dunbar, R. I. M. (1992). Neocortex size as a constraint on group size in primates. *Journal of Human Evolution*, 22(6), 469–493. https://doi.org/10.1016/0047-2484(92)90081-J

Dunbar, R. I. M. (1998). *Grooming, gossip, and the evolution of language*. Harvard University Press.

Edwards, C., Allan, R., Marzo, N., Wynfield, T., & Hicks, R. (2023). The use of emotionally focused therapy with polyamorous relationships. *Family Process*, 62(4), 1362–1376. https://doi.org/10.1111/famp.12934

Evces, M. R. (2015). What is vicarious trauma? In G. Quitangon & M. R. Evces (Eds.), *Vicarious trauma and disaster mental health: Understanding risks and promoting resilience* (pp. 9–23). Routledge.

Felitti, V. J., Anda, R. F., Nordenberg, D., Williamson, D. F., Spitz, A. M., Edwards, V., Koss, M. P., & Marks, J. S. (1998). Relationship of childhood abuse and household dysfunction to many of the leading causes of death in adults: The Adverse Childhood Experiences (ACE) Study. *American Journal of Preventive Medicine*, 14(4), 245–258. https://doi.org/10.1016/S0749-3797(98)00017-8

Fern, J. (2020). *Polysecure: Attachment, Trauma and Consensual Nonmonogamy*. Thorntree Press.

Fox, J. G. (2020). Recovery, interrupted: The Zeigarnik effect in EMDR therapy and the adaptive information processing model. *Journal of EMDR Practice & Research*, 14(3), 175–185.

Fox, M. J. (2012, March 29). Michael J. Fox at 50: "I'm still happy." *The Palm Beach Post*. www.palmbeachpost.com/story/entertainment/human-interest/2012/03/29/michael-j-fox-at-50/7467199007

Fraley, R. C., Gillath, O., & Deboeck, P. R. (2021). Do life events lead to enduring changes in adult attachment styles? A naturalistic longitudinal investigation. *Journal of Personality and Social Psychology*, 120(6), 1567–1606. https://doi.org/10.1037/pspi0000326

Freyd, J. J. (2021). *What is a betrayal trauma? What is betrayal trauma theory?* http://pages.uoregon.edu/dynamic/jjf/defineBT.html

Goerlich, S. (2023). *With sprinkles on top: Everything vanilla people and their kinky partners need to know to communicate, explore, and connect*. Sounds True.

Goleman, D. (1995). *Emotional intelligence: Why it can matter more than IQ*. Bantam Books.

Gordon, T. (1970). *Parent effectiveness training: The no-lose program for raising responsible children.* Wyden Books.

Gottman, J. M., & Silver, N. (2012). *What makes love last? How to build trust and avoid betrayal.* Simon & Schuster.

Hardy, J. W., & Easton, D. (2017). *The ethical slut: A practical guide to polyamory, open relationships, and other freedoms in sex and love* (3rd ed.). Ten Speed Press.

Hari, J. (2015, July). *Everything you think you know about addiction is wrong* [Video]. TED Conferences. www.ted.com/talks/johann_hari_everything_you_think_you_know_about_addiction_is_wrong

Herman, J. L. (1992). *Trauma and recovery: The aftermath of violence: From domestic abuse to political terror.* Basic Books.

Hoffman-Fox, D. (2017). *You and your gender identity: A guide to discovery.* Differential Publishing.

Hollenbeck, C., & Steffens, B. (2024). Betrayal trauma anger: Clinical implications for therapeutic treatment based on the sexually betrayed partner's experience related to anger after intimate betrayal. *Journal of Sex & Marital Therapy, 50*(4), 456–467. https://doi.org/10.1080/00926 23X.2024.2306940

Johnson, J., & Noire, K. (2021). *Trauma, drama, and kink* [Live Workshop]. Modern Sex Therapy Institutes.

Johnson, S. M. (2004). *The practice of emotionally focused couple therapy: Creating connection* (2nd ed.). Brunner-Routledge.

Johnson, S. M. (2008). *Hold me tight: Seven conversations for a lifetime of love.* Little, Brown.

Jules, B. N., O'Connor, V. L., & Langhinrichsen-Rohling, J. (2023). Judgments of event centrality as predictors of post-traumatic growth and post-traumatic stress after infidelity: The moderating effect of relationship form. *Trauma Care, 3*(4), 237–250. https://doi.org/10.3390/traumacare3040021

Kübler-Ross, E. (1969). *On death and dying.* Macmillan.

Laaser, M., & Laaser, D. (2017). *Hula Hoop Health: The stages of relational development.* https://store.faithfulandtrue.com/products/hula-hoop-health-pdf

Levine, D. (2022). Neuroscience of emotion, cognition, and decision making: A review. *ESMED Medical Review Archives, 10*(3), 125–134. https://esmed.org/MRA/mra/article/download/2869/193546185

Lipps, T. (1903). Ästhetik: Psychologie des Schönen und der Kunst [Aesthetics: Psychology of beauty and art]. Engelmann.

Lonergan, M., Brunet, A., Rivest-Beauregard, M., & Groleau, D. (2021). Is romantic partner betrayal a form of traumatic experience? A qualitative study. *Stress and Health, 37*(1), 19–31. https://doi.org/10.1002/smi.2968

Luft, J., & Ingham, H. (1955). The Johari window: A graphic model for interpersonal relations. *Proceedings of the Western Training Laboratory in Group Development.* University of California, Los Angeles.

Main, M., & Solomon, J. (1986). Discovery of a new, insecure-disorganized/disoriented attachment pattern. In T. B. Brazelton & M. W. Yogman (Eds.), *Affective development in infancy* (pp. 95–124). Ablex Publishing.

Marín, R., Christensen, A., & Atkins, D. (2014). Infidelity and behavioral couple therapy: Relationship outcomes over 5 years following therapy. *Couple and Family Psychology: Research and Practice, 3*(1), 1–12. https://doi.org/10.1037/cfp0000012

Maslow, A. H. (1943). A theory of human motivation. *Psychological Review, 50*(4), 370–396.

Mauritz, M. W., Goossens, P. J. J., Draijer, N., & van Achterberg, T. (2013). Prevalence of interpersonal trauma exposure and trauma-related disorders in severe mental illness. *European Journal of Psychotraumatology, 4*(1), 19985. https://doi.org/10.3402/ejpt.v4i0.19985

Mellody, P., Miller, A. W., & Miller, J. K. (1989). *Facing codependence: What it is, where it comes from, how it sabotages our lives*. Harper & Row.

Merriam-Webster. (n.d.-a). Abuse. In *Merriam-Webster.com dictionary*. www.merriam-webster.com/dictionary/abuse

Merriam-Webster. (n.d.-b). Pleasure. In *Merriam-Webster.com dictionary*. www.merriam-webster.com/dictionary/pleasure

Merriam-Webster. (n.d.-c). Accountability. In *Merriam-Webster.com dictionary*. www.merriam-webster.com/dictionary/accountability

Merriam-Webster. (n.d.-d). Deception. In *Merriam-Webster.com dictionary*. www.merriam-webster.com/dictionary/deception

Meyer, S. (2005). *Twilight*. Little, Brown and Company.

Minuchin, S. (1974). *Families and family therapy*. Harvard University Press.

Minwalla, O. (2021). *The secret sexual basement: The traumatic impacts of deceptive sexuality on the intimate partner and relationship* (White paper, February, revised November). The Institute for Sexual Health.

Murray, M. (2021). *The Murray method: Creating wholeness beyond trauma, abuse, neglect, and addiction*. Vivo Publications.

Nagoski, E. (2016, January). *Confidence and joy are the keys to a great sex life* [Video]. TEDx University of Nevada. www.ted.com/talks/emily_nagoski_confidence_and_joy_are_the_keys_to_a_great_sex_life

Nagoski, E. (2018, April). *The truth about unwanted arousal* [Video]. TED Conferences. www.ted.com/talks/emily_nagoski_the_truth_about_unwanted_arousal

Nagoski, E. (2021). *Come as you are: Revised and updated: The surprising new science that will transform your sex life*. Simon & Schuster.

Nagoski, E. (2024). *Come together: The science (and art!) of creating lasting sexual connections*. Ballantine Books.

Neff, K. (2011). *Self-compassion: Stop beating yourself up and leave insecurity behind*. William Morrow.

Nightingale, M., Awosan, C. I., & Stavrianopoulos, K. (2019). Emotionally focused therapy: A culturally sensitive approach for African American heterosexual couples. *Journal of Family Psychotherapy, 30*(3), 221–244. https://doi.org/10.1080/08975353.2019.1666497

Pietrzykowski, T., & Smilowska, K. (2021). The reality of informed consent: Empirical studies on patient comprehension – Systematic review. *Trials, 22*(1), 57. https://doi.org/10.1186/s13063-020-04969-w

Plutchik, R. (2001). The nature of emotions: Human emotions have deep evolutionary roots, a fact that may explain their complexity and provide tools for clinical practice. *American Scientist, 89*(4), 344–350.

Rape, Abuse & Incest National Network (RAINN). (n.d.). Perpetrators of sexual violence: Statistics. *RAINN*. www.rainn.org/statistics/perpetrators-sexual-violence

Riordan, J. P. (2022). Dyadic trauma and attachment: A monozygotic twin study assessing the efficacy of Somatic Experiencing®. *Journal of Applied Neurosciences, 1*(1), a3.

Rogers, C. R. (1957). The necessary and sufficient conditions of therapeutic personality change. *Journal of Consulting Psychology, 21*(2), 95–103. https://doi.org/10.1037/h0045357

Rokach, A., & Chan, S. (2023). Love and infidelity: Causes and consequences. *International Journal of Environmental Research and Public Health*, 20(5), 3904.

Satir, V. (1964). *Conjoint family therapy: A guide to theory and technique*. Science and Behavior Books.

Siegel, R. (2019). Therapists who address O.C.S.B. In J. C. Wadley & R. Siegel (Eds.), *The art of sex therapy supervision*. Routledge.

Stavrova, O., Pronk, T., & Denissen, J. (2023). Estranged and unhappy? Examining the dynamics of personal and relationship well-being surrounding infidelity. *Psychological Science*, 34(2), 143–169. https://doi.org/10.1177/09567976221116892

Steffens, B., & Rennie, R. (2006). The traumatic nature of disclosure for wives of sexual addicts. *Journal of Sexual Health & Compulsivity*, 13(2–3), 247–267.

Substance Abuse and Mental Health Services Administration (SAMHSA). (2024, November 8). *Trauma and violence*. US Department of Health and Human Services. www.samhsa.gov/mental-health/trauma-violence

Tirone, V., Orlowska, D., Lofgreen, A. M., Blais, R. K., Stevens, N. R., Klassen, B., Held, P., & Zalta, A. K. (2021). The association between social support and posttraumatic stress symptoms among survivors of betrayal trauma: A meta-analysis. *European Journal of Psychotraumatology*, 12(1). https://doi.org/10.1080/20008198.2021.1883925

Titchener, E. B. (1909). *Lectures on the experimental psychology of the thought-processes*. Macmillan.

Tracy, J. L., & Randles, D. (2011). Four models of basic emotions: A review of current debates. *Emotion Review*, 3(4), 397–405. https://doi.org/10.1177/1754073911410747

Warach, B., & Josephs, L. (2021). The aftershocks of infidelity: A review of infidelity-based attachment trauma. *Sexual and Relationship Therapy*, 36(1), 68–90. https://doi.org/10.1080/14681994.2019.1577961

Wegscheider-Cruse, S. (1981). *Another chance: Hope and health for the alcoholic family*. Science and Behavior Books.

World Health Organization. (n.d.). *Sexual health*. World Health Organization. www.who.int/teams/sexual-and-reproductive-health-and-research-(srh)/areas-of-work/sexual-health

Index

Note: *Italic* page numbers refer to figures.

For Product Safety Concerns and Information please contact our EU
representative GPSR@taylorandfrancis.com
Taylor & Francis Verlag GmbH, Kaufingerstraße 24, 80331 München, Germany